the CUPS diet

Dr. Mascaro's Portion Control
to Losing Weight is Effective and Easy
by Dr. Jimmy R. Mascaro
Copyright 2014

FIRST EDITION
ISBN-13: 978-1492724032
ISBN-10: 1492724033
V101714

Published by

MASCARO HEALTH, INC.

06/10/13

www.thecupsdiet.com

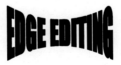

2505 SW Seabrook Avenue
Suite 1
Topeka, KS 66614
1-785-430-8618
edgeediting8@gmail.com

USERS of the CUPS diet®

the CUPS diet® continues to grow in popularity, as is reflected by our rapidly expanding user base. The map below shows the domestic user distribution as of this printing. These results will be regularly updated in the eBook and in any future printings.

There are now users in 44 **states**; AK, AL, AR, AZ, CA, CO, CT, FL, GA, HI, IA, IL, IN, KS, LA, MA, MD, ME, MI, MN, MO, MS, NB, NC, ND, NH, NJ, NM, NV, NY, OH, OK, OR, PA, SC, SD, TN, TX, UT, VA, WA, WI, WV, and WY.

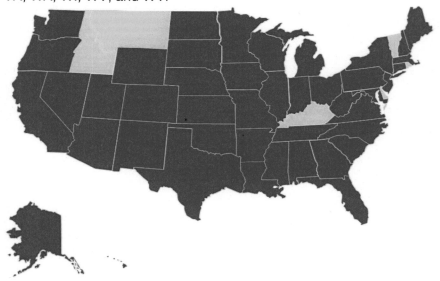

the CUPS diet® - It works!!!

INTERNATIONAL USERS of the CUPS diet®

the CUPS diet® continues to grow in popularity internationally also, as is reflected by our rapidly expanding user base. The map below shows the user distribution as of this printing. These results will be regularly updated in the eBook and in any future printings.

Now with users in 10 **countries** (including territories); Argentina, Australia, Canada, Costa Rica, Germany, Ireland, Switzerland, United Arab Emirates, United Kingdom, U.S.A., and the U.S. Virgin Islands.

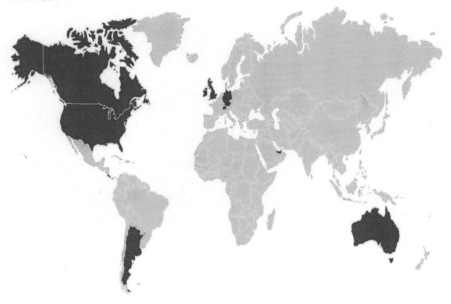

the CUPS diet® - It works!!!

WEIGHT LOSS RESULTS

Listed below are our top ten users in total weight loss and the top four users in most weight lost in the first three weeks. These results will be regularly updated in the eBook and in any future book printings.

The "Top 10" in total weight loss

1. 125.0 lbs. (56.7kg) by MM
2. 79.0 lbs. (35.8kg) by LG
3. 66.9 lbs. (30.3kg) by WR
4. 65.8 lbs. (29.8kg) by CS
5. 50.0 lbs. (22.7kg) by LB
6. 46.0 lbs. (20.9kg) by BG
7. 45.0 lbs. (20.4kg) by SK & KV
8. 44.0 lbs. (20.0kg) by AS
9. 39.2 lbs. (17.8kg) by CI
10. 39.0 lbs. (17.7kg) by LJ & EJ

The "Top 4 in under 4" for weight lost in 3 weeks

1. 26.0 pounds (11.8kg) by LG in less than 4 weeks
2. 17.0 pounds (07.7kg) by BB in less than 4 weeks
3. 16.5 pounds (07.5kg) by EJ in less than 4 weeks
4. 15.3 pounds (07.0kg) by CS in less than 4 weeks

the CUPS diet® - It works!!!

SUCCESS STORIES

A GREAT DIET

"This has been a great diet for me ... With it (**the CUPS diet®**) I can actually go out and eat and enjoy the foods I love from time to time and still continue to lose weight. Combined with my workout program I have lost more weight and I have been able to keep it off more successfully than I ever had in the past."

Matt (page 29) – Des Moines, Iowa, lost 125 lbs. (56.7kg)

BEST PROGRAM OUT THERE

"This has been a fabulous diet. I am feeling great about it. It is the best program out there!"

Carla - Bloomfield, Iowa, lost 65.8 lbs. (29.8kg)

IT'S a NEW LIFE

"I started following **the CUPS diet®** and I am eating foods I enjoy, in controlled portions. I drink a lot of water and get a good deal of exercise, mostly walking. Not only have I lost a lot of weight, but my blood sugar has dropped from critical to normal and my attitude is much more positive.

Lee – Lawrence, Kansas, lost 79 lbs. (35.8kg)

ENERGY and HEALTH HAVE IMPROVED

"When I started, my evening blood sugars ran in the 300's and I took 55 units of Lantos insulin. I found the diet to be very easy and I could eat whatever I wanted. After a few short weeks my evening blood sugars dropped to the low 200s and after only six weeks they were between 134-180 and my Lantos dropped to 0-25 units a day. My energy and health have improved so much. I've had gastric bypass surgery in the 1970's and that didn't work. I tried many diets and couldn't stay on them because of the restrictions they imposed, but now I am able to eat whatever I want and control how much. I have had a hip replacement and my physical activity is limited but I am still able to lose weight."

Kevin - Ottumwa, Iowa, lost 44 lbs. (20kg)

VERY EASY ... VERY EFFECTIVE

"I would recommend **the CUPS diet®** to anyone wanting to lose weight. It is very easy to stick with, and very effective. It is the #1 diet in my opinion."

Larry (page 37) - Albia, Iowa, lost 39 lbs. (17.7kg)

EATING FOODS I LOVE

"Thanks ... eating foods I love."

Renee - Ottumwa, Iowa, lost 29.5 lbs. (13.4kg)

YOUR PROGRAM is WORKING FINE

"I am doing well. Your program is working just fine with my cardiac rehab and I am losing weight. Thank you, thank you, thank you!"

Beth - Ottumwa, Iowa, lost 17 lbs. (7.7kg)

IT FEELS GOOD to be SUCCEEDING

"Your plan (**the CUPS diet®**) is much more realistic than most anything on the market. It is the only thing I have stuck to for more than a week .... It feels good to be succeeding! ... I am very excited to be on this path ... I could not remember what it felt like to be thin and healthy ... it is getting easier every day!"

Jamie - Seattle, Washington, lost 28 lbs. (12.7kg)

LUCKIEST PERSON in the WORLD

"I was facing multiple joint replacements and was overweight, very close to obesity. My orthopedist recommended that I lose a significant amount of weight prior to the procedures. I decided on **the CUPS diet®**, and it did the job for me and then some. My new right knee simply would have been under too much strain if I hadn't lost weight. Now I am scheduled to have my left knee replaced. Having done so in such a safe and sane manner for my first surgery assured me that there would be no unnecessary complications this time. I have gotten more exercise this time around and am even more confident before going into my second surgery. Dr. Mascaro, your diet has literally been a life saver for me."

Ellen - Topeka, Kansas, lost 39 lbs. (17.7kg)

I RECOMMEND it to EVERYBODY

"I am losing weight and I am keeping it off, unlike my previous weight loss attempts. I now am able to be more in control of my eating habits, and I eat whatever I want, however in appropriate portions. That is something I could never do before with any of the other diets I have tried. I am very comfortable with this diet and I would highly recommend it to everybody. Thank you Dr. Mascaro for inventing **the CUPS diet®**. You are awesome!!!"

Veronika – Cedar Rapids, Iowa, lost 20 lbs. (9.1kg)

LIFE-LONG CHANGE

"Things are going so well and I am quite content on this program (**the CUPS diet®**). I am so amazed that it is working so well in terms of satisfaction and in weight loss. Other diets will tell you that you have to completely stop eating the foods that you crave in order to stop the craving. Not true. My cravings are very much under control because I know that I can have it if I want it ... I want to tell you how HAPPY I am to be still sticking with this diet. It is a life-long change. To be sticking with this over weekends and through the holidays is an absolute first ... I think, that in terms of longevity, this plan works best for me."

Susan - Cedar Rapids, Iowa, lost 24 lbs. (10.9kg)

I WAS LOSING WEIGHT

"Someone asked if I was losing weight, that's a big thing."

Barb - Des Moines, Iowa, lost 28 lbs. (12.7kg)

NOT FEELING HUNGRY

"I am simply not feeling hungry on this diet."

Chris - Seattle, Washington, lost 25.5 lbs. (11.6kg)

EVEN I LOST WEIGHT

"I am not known for my self-discipline, but when I gained twenty pounds over the course of a couple of months, I decided to take action. I started **the CUPS**

diet® and during the next nine weeks lost 23.5 pounds. My conclusion: feeling better was sure better than feeling lazy."

Roger – Topeka, Kansas, lost 37 lbs. (16.7kg)

I CAN EAT ANYTHING
"I can eat anything on **the CUPS diet**®."

Jessie - Cedar Rapids, Iowa, lost 12 lbs. (5.4kg)

BEST DIET I HAVE EVER BEEN ON
" ... **the CUPS diet**® is the best diet I have ever been on. I have not been hungry and I am seeing results; putting clothes on I have not worn for years, and I am getting closer to my goal ... I thought my metabolism had quit working ... however by portion control and the choices I make, it works GREAT!!!"

Sandy - Ollie, Iowa, lost 22 lbs. (10kg)

EASY to STAY ON
"I found that **the CUPS diet**® was pretty easy to stay on and I found a way to increase my calcium intake by eating more broccoli and also by placing a slice of cheese on my veggies. It was a very good alternative for me instead of drinking several glasses of milk every day."

Kitley – Ankeny, Iowa, lost 24 lbs. (10.9kg)

EASY PLAN to FOLLOW
"I have been overweight most of my adult life and on several diets. On **the CUPS diet**® you do not feel deprived of your favorite foods and it is an easy plan to follow at home or when you are eating out. There are no calories or carbs to count and you are not tied down with weighing and measuring everything."

Rosemary - Eddyville, Iowa, lost 34 lbs. (15.4kg)

SPECIAL NOTE

Before starting on **the CUPS diet**® *it is very important that you assess your current weight associated health risks (page 33) and also carefully consider your weight loss goals and expectations.*

Be sure to consult with your doctor to determine whether the state of your health warrants altering your dietary habits by reducing your caloric intake before you start on this or any diet.

Seek advice from your doctor as to whether you can safely increase your level of physical activity (page 89) to help achieve your weight loss goals. **the CUPS diet**® *is for men and women (non-pregnant) age 18 and older.*

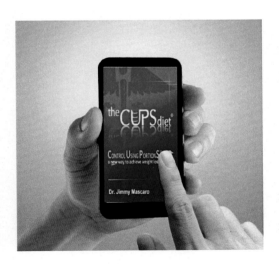

TABLE of CONTENTS

QUICK START: Go to **CHAPTER SIX,**
and then be sure to review **CHAPTERS SEVEN-TEN.**

USERS of the CUPS diet®	02
INTERNATIONAL USERS of the CUPS diet®	03
WEIGHT LOSS RESULTS	04
SUCCESS STORIES	05
DEDICATION and ACKNOWLEDGEMENTS	14
INTRODUCTION	15
ABOUT Dr. MASCARO	16
the CUPS diet® BOOK(s)	18
TERMS USED in this BOOK	22
..... Adjusted Individual Measurement (AIM)	22
..... Basal Metabolic Rate (BMR)	22
..... Body Mass Index (BMI)	22
..... Control Using PortionS™ (CUPS)	22
..... Count times 2 [**Cx2**]	22
..... COUPLE of CUPS	23
..... CUP for CUP vegetables [**C/C**]	23
..... First Fruits Free [**FFF**]	23
CHAPTER ONE - DEVELOPMENT of **the CUPS diet®**	25
CHAPTER TWO - OBESITY, A CHRONIC DISEASE	30
..... Body Mass Index (BMI)	31
..... Epidemic Proportions	32
..... Weight Associated Health Risk	32
..... Disease Risks Based on BMI	33
..... We Get What We Pay For	34
CHAPTER THREE - THE IDEAL WEIGHT	35
..... Ideal Weight and Normal Weight and Healthy Weight	36
..... Desired Weight and Motivation	37
.... "Success Points"	38

TABLE of CONTENTS

CHAPTER FOUR - FUNCTIONAL vs. FAD DIETS	39
CHAPTER FIVE - HOW **the CUPS diet®** WORKS	42
..... Control Using PortionS™ (CUPS)	42
..... Portion vs. Serving	42
..... Basal Metabolic Rate (BMR)	43
..... Adjusted Individual Measurement (**AIM**)	44
..... Companion Website (www.thecupsdiet.com)	45
CHAPTER SIX - HOW MUCH CAN I EAT?	46
..... Adjusted Individual Measurement (**AIM**)	46
CHAPTER SEVEN - USING **the CUPS diet®**	49
..... Directions for Daily Use	50
CHAPTER EIGHT - ESTIMATING PORTIONS	57
..... Estimating Food Volume	57
.... LARGE Portions	59
..... Equivalents	61
..... CUPS Approximation Examples (photo)	62
CHAPTER NINE - FOOD GROUPS and CATEGORIES	63
..... the five Food Groups	63
.... 1. Vegetables	63
.... 2. Fruits	64
.... 3. Dairy Products	64
.... 4. Grains	64
.... 5. Meats	65
..... the five Special Food Categories	65
.... 1. Count times 2 [**Cx2**]	65
.... 2. CUPS for CUP vegetables [**C/C**]	67
.... 3. First Fruits Free [**FFF**]	67
.... 4. Meats [**M**]	68
.... 5. NO count foods and beverages [**Ø**]	69
CHAPTER TEN – MEALS and SNACKS and WATER	71
..... Meals	71
.... Breakfast	71
.... Example of a Breakfast	72

TABLE of CONTENTS

..... Snacks	73
..... Water	73
..... Daily Menu "SAMPLE" (1 of 2)	74
CHAPTER ELEVEN – CONDIMENTS	79
..... Creams [**Cx2**] and Dairy [**Cx2**] – LFP (Low Fat Preferred)	80
..... Oils [**Cx2**] and Fats [**Cx2**] – LFP	80
..... Sauces	80
..... Spices and Herbs [**Ø**]	80
..... Spreads and Toppings - LFP	81
..... Sugars [**Cx2**] and Syrups [**Cx2**] – low calorie preferred	81
CHAPTER TWELVE - TIPS FOR LOSING WEIGHT	82
APPENDIX I - FACTORS AFFECTING the BMR	85
APPENDIX II - EXAMPLES of HEALTHY MEALS	90
APPENDIX III - FOOD APPROXIMATIONS in CUPS	117
..... Beverages	118
.... Alcohol	118
.... Coffee [**Ø**] and Tea [**Ø**]	119
.... Juice and Milk	120
.... Protein and Soda and Water [**Ø**]	121
..... Breads and Grains	122
..... Dairy (1 of 2)	123
..... Desserts [**Cx2**] and Sweets [**Cx2**]	124
..... Fast Foods	126
.... Burger King (1 of 3)	126
.... Dairy Queen (1 of 2)	129
.... KFC (1 of 3)	131
.... McDonald's (1 of 2)	134
.... Panda Express (1 of 2)	136
.... Pizza Hut	138
.... Subway	139
.... Taco Bell (1 of 2)	140
.... Wendy's (1 of 2)	142
.... White Castle and Wingstop	144

TABLE of CONTENTS

..... Fruits [**FFF**] - Fresh Fruits (1 of 5) — 145
..... Fruits - (non-fresh) and Fruit Products — 150
..... Meats [**M**] (1 of 2) — 151
..... Nuts [**Cx2**] and Seeds [**Cx2**] — 153
..... Pizza — 154
..... Sandwiches — 155
..... Snack Foods and Chips — 155
..... Snacks (1 of 2) — 156
..... Vegetables – **NO** count vegetables [**Ø**] (1 of 3) — 158
..... The "CUP for CUP" vegetables [**C/C**] — 161
..... From the **CUP**board – Mascaro Family Recipes — 162
.... Boursin Stuffed Mushrooms — 164
.... Bread (no-knead) — 166
.... Caesar Salad — 168
.... Chicken Pot Pie — 170
.... Crab Cakes — 172
.... Crusted Pork Chops — 174
.... Double Pie Crust — 176
.... Flan — 178
.... Grilled Pita Flat Bread Pizza — 180
.... Italian Roasted Potatoes — 182
.... Mediterranean Potato Salad — 184
.... Morir Soñando — 186
.... Salsa — 188
.... Spinach Dip — 190
.... Taco Rico — 192
..... Final Comments — 194
..... Index — 195

DEDICATION

I dedicate this book to my beautiful wife and best friend, Hilda. Her input and suggestions were invaluable in making **the CUPS diet®** the unique and innovative work that it is. I am grateful for her patience and support whenever I said I had to work on "the book".

ACKNOWLEDGEMENTS

I want to thank my family, including my mother Patty and my father Angelo, my children Matt, Angie, Andrea, and Alex for their ideas and suggestions, as well as their support and encouragement.

I also want to thank my editor Roger Jones, my website team Global Reach Internet Productions of Ames, Iowa, Beth Harrington at bDesign Photography in Ottumwa, Iowa, who handled the graphic design of the book cover, and last, but not least, PerLa Nancy González Salazar, a Registered Dietician from Monterrey, Nuevo León, Mexico, who helped provide the healthy meal examples (page 90).

INTRODUCTION

An increasing number of people worldwide now struggle with weight problems. Approximately 50% of adults are overweight or obese in about half of the world's developed countries. In the United States over two thirds of the adult population is overweight; with more than one third meeting the criteria for obesity.

Predictably, as the rates of being overweight or obese increase, the diet book market continues to expand as well.

" **... With some 38,000 diet books in print - and 2,500 new ones hitting the shelves every year - not to mention magazines trumpeting the ultimate new fad diet in every monthly issue, there's plenty to choose from ... "** *http://men.webmd.com/guide/diet-plans-men*

Some diet books and weight loss plans are medically sound. However many can be impractical and unrealistic, while a few are basically unhealthy or even potentially dangerous. The sheer number of books available that for the most part aren't effective is strong evidence that it is time to take a different approach. An approach that works!

For an easy, healthy, and common sense way to lose weight, use **the CUPS diet**®. I wish you the best as you lose weight, reduce health risks, and enjoy a higher state of physical and mental well-being.

Sincerely,

Dr. Mascaro

ABOUT Dr. MASCARO

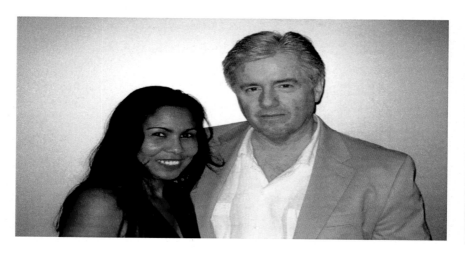

Dr. Jimmy R. Mascaro, D.O., is an adult psychiatrist licensed in the states of New York and Iowa. He is the creator and author of **the CUPS diet®** as well as the administrator of the website, www.thecupsdiet.com (page 23).

Dr. Mascaro maintains a clinical practice at the Southern Iowa Mental Health Center in Ottumwa, Iowa, where he provides psychiatric services for adults. His wife, Dr. Hilda M. Mascaro, M.D., a child and adolescent psychiatrist licensed in New York and Iowa, provides psychiatric services for children and Spanish speaking patients. Both utilize on-site and telepsychiatric care.

After receiving his undergraduate degree (Bachelor of Science), with a major in Psychology from Iowa State University in Ames, Iowa, Dr. Mascaro attended medical school at Des Moines University in Des Moines, Iowa, where he graduated with a Doctor of Osteopathic Medicine degree. His residency in Psychiatry was at the University of Iowa Hospitals and Clinics in Iowa City, Iowa.

Dr. Mascaro has also served as the Medical Director for Adult Psychiatric Medicine at Ottumwa Regional Health Center, and as an Adjunct Clinical Instructor of Psychiatry for Des Moines University.

Dr. Mascaro currently resides in New York and routinely returns to his home state of Iowa.

In December, 2003, Dr. Mascaro began developing an easier and more practical way (using portion control) to achieve and maintain weight loss. The result was **the CUPS diet®**.

Dr. Mascaro is a member of the following professional associations, societies, and organizations:

American Diabetes Association, *Alexandria, Virginia*
American Medical Association, *Chicago, Illinois*
American Psychiatric Association, *Arlington, Virginia*
American Society for Nutrition, *Bethesda, Maryland*
Dominican Medical Association, Inc. , *New York, New York*
Iowa Psychiatric Society, *Des Moines, Iowa*
Obesity Action Coalition, *Tampa, Florida*
The Obesity Society, *Silver Spring, Maryland*

the CUPS diet® BOOK(s)

the CUPS diet® book and eBook version have been developed because this weight loss method has proven so effective for me and many, many others, including my patients and numerous subscribers to www.thecupsdiet.com.

COMPANION WEBSITE

UPDATEABLE

PORTABLE AND CONVENIENT

SUPPORT

Companion website – with this book you will receive **FREE** website access (page 23), a benefit available to those purchasing this book and is perhaps the most important tool that we are offering.

Very few diet programs have websites as their backbone, and if they do, it is unlikely that their utility is as great as that offered at www.thecupsdiet.com. At our site you are offered a full range of services, from assistance in getting started to daily monitoring of your progress on the path toward a healthy and sustainable ideal weight.

Updateable – as relevant research or advice on nutrition and weight loss becomes available, updates will be made to **the CUPS diet®** companion website, eBook and future printings. To get the latest version of **the CUPS diet®** eBook go to your Amazon.com account and select "Manage Your Kindle". Make sure you select the option to have your eBooks updated automatically.

Then select "BOOKS" on the left side. Search for "the CUPS diet" and when you have it select the "ACTIONS" tab that is on on the right. Choose "DELIVER TO MY"...and choose your device in the drop down menu. All updates will be announced through FACEBOOK and will then be noted at the website under in FAQS, www.thecupsdiet.com/index.cfm?action=cFAQs.list, under "eBook Update". You should then check the website or FACEBOOK on a weekly basis to be sure you have the latest of **the CUPS diet®**. If this update does not work, contact Kindle support.

Portable – its convenience cannot be overstated. You can now take your diet plan with you everywhere you go as you lose weight in any setting with website (page 23) access and your eBook/book. This is particularly true in the case of the Kindle and any Apple or Android device or smartphone.

Support – user support is available should you have any questions, comments, or suggestions. Send an email to me, at drmascaro@thecupsdiet.com or visit www.thecupsdiet.com and select "contact" in the upper right hand corner and send me a message. I want your experience with **the CUPS diet®** to be positive and I want it to meet your needs. So, let ME work personally for you and assist you with motivation and encouragement as well as addressing any questions or concerns that may arise regarding your specific progress.

the CUPS diet® has a user support forum on FACEBOOK. Select "Like" **the CUPS diet®** page and you will be able to discuss user support, motivation, weight loss tips, weight loss results, nutrition, and exercise. The forum can also be used to evaluate the opinions of others, as well as for asking questions, conducting a poll, or simply keeping in touch with other users of **the CUPS diet®**.

Should you choose to purchase the eBook version and the published version of **the CUPS diet®**, you will have the ultimate weight loss and maintenance plan always at your fingertips.

eBOOK ADVANTAGES

In addition to being able to "**Go to...**" sections or chapters within **the CUPS diet®** eBook, you will also find a fully interactive TABLE of CONTENTS and hyperlinks (**blue** or underlined terms) referring to key words or chapters. These will prove to be handy tools which allow you to search within the book with little effort. To return to the previous page you were reading, press the "go BACK" arrow (←) on the Options Bar for your eReader.

Next are a few tips on optimal reading settings for various eReaders, smartphones, and computers.

Optimal eBook Reading Settings	
Portrait (best)	Size: 3 – 7
Landscape	Size: 4 – 11
Font	Helvetica (best), Georgia, Arial
Margins	Small
Words per Line	Maximum
Line Spacing	Small
Text-to-Speech	On or Off

Align your tables so that most will fit evenly on each page. Larger or smaller text sizes may be used; however larger sizes may cause the text or the tables to be split between pages. Adjust your text size accordingly or based upon your own personal preferences (KINDLE for PC, HTML or PDF for Smashwords.com).

Following are some suggested text sizes and settings for a number of popular eReaders.

ANDROID Smartphone
Portrait Size: 4th largest
Landscape Size: 10th largest

APPLE iPad
Portrait Size: 4th - 5th largest

APPLE iPhone 4
Portrait Size: 3rd largest
Landscape Size: 10th largest

APPLE iPhone 5
Portrait Size: 2nd – 4th largest
Landscape Size: 8th - 9th largest
Font: Helvetica
Line Spacing: small

KINDLE Keyboard
Portrait Size: 4th largest
Landscape Size: 4th largest
Typeface: regular
Line Spacing: small
Words per Line: default

KINDLE Fire
Portrait Size: 4th largest

KINDLE Fire HD
Portrait Size: #6
Font: Helvetica
Line Spacing: small
Margins: narrow

KINDLE Fire HD 8.9
Portrait & Landscape Size: #7
Font: Helvetica
Line Spacing: small
Margins: narrow

KINDLE Paperwhite
Portrait Size: 4th largest from left
Font: Helvetica
Line Spacing: small
Margins: narrow

KINDLE for PC
Portrait Size: 4th - 8th largest
Two Columns: 4th - 5th largest

TERMS USED in this BOOK

Adjusted Individual Measurement (AIM)

is the amount of food that an individual "aims" at eating in a typical day in order to lose weight at a consistent and healthy rate. **the CUPS diet®** utilizes an innovative system of monitoring food consumption, based on food volume using measuring cup increments (page 44).

To get your initial **AIM** go to Chapter SIX (page 46).

Basal Metabolic Rate (BMR)

is the minimum caloric intake needed to sustain basic bodily functions such as respiration, the cardiovascular system, and body temperature maintenance, to name a few (page 43).

Body Mass Index (BMI)

is a standard method (page 31) for estimating whether an individual may be considered overweight or obese, and thus revealing any weight associated health risks (page 33).

Control Using PortionS™ (CUPS)

is the method of weight management (losing, gaining, or maintaining) based on portion control achieved by an accurate monitoring of food (page 42).

Count times 2 [Cx2]

is a SPECIAL FOOD CATEGORY of foods (page 65), that, because of the uniqueness of their nutritional composition (calories, fats, carbohydrates, cholesterol, sugars, etc.), are counted twice.

COUPLE of CUPS

is a "wellness concept" (page 82) that aids in meal planning and weight loss by providing intake recommendations for an average day from the different FOOD GROUPS (page 63).

CUP for CUP vegetables [C/C]

is a SPECIAL FOOD CATEGORY comprised of vegetables that count as estimated, that is, cup for cup, when determining your daily food intake. All other vegetables do not count toward your AIM.

First Fruits Free [FFF]

is a SPECIAL FOOD CATEGORY of fresh fruits (page 67). Because of their nutritional and health benefits, these are counted after intake exceeds 2 cups.

When using **the CUPS diet®** it will never be necessary to use any formulas or perform any calculations to determine your AIM, BMI, or BMR. All of these will be calculated for you at the website.

Obtaining your FREE Website Access
1. Visit www.thecupsdiet.com and select the blue Book Access tab
2. Enter the access information that is requested, which includes:
.... Source of your book purchase and order or receipt number
.... Type of eReader, tablet, smartphone, or computer
.... Email, password, name, country, and state
.... Current and desired weight (lbs.), height, date of birth, gender
3. Select Sign Up and enter your email, password, and then Sign In
4. Follow steps 6-9 found on page 50 on using **the CUPS diet®**

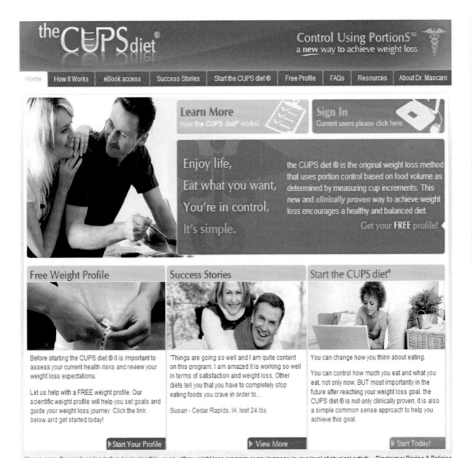

Screenshot *"**HOMEPAGE**" from the companion website, www.thecupsdiet.com*

CHAPTER ONE

DEVELOPMENT of the CUPS diet®

In December, 2003, after several unsuccessful attempts at losing weight by trying a variety of diet schemes, I realized that I had only been successful in losing my patience and not in losing my weight. This personal experience of being unable to lose weight through the use of methods devised by others convinced me that it was time to develop an easier and more effective way to achieve weight loss. As I had battled weight problems since my youth and had evaluated many of the so-called road maps to the land of "thin", I was already aware of the fact that many diet plans have inherent flaws.

These flaws make many diet plans unacceptable as effective tools for sustained and healthy weight loss. Among these weaknesses and shortcomings are:

Many diets .....
..... are not beneficial to overall health
..... do not consider psychological aspects
..... may call for investment in costly foods
..... ask that you purchase supplements
..... won't let you enjoy favorite foods
..... often require extensive meal planning
..... are not family-friendly and do not allow for dining out
..... involve tedious measuring of food
..... may require complex food counting
..... often use complicated recordkeeping
..... are too restrictive to follow long-term

It became clear to me that an effective and sustainable diet would allow me to eat foods I enjoyed without imposing unreasonable restrictions. I felt that a very simple method of monitoring food intake was necessary. This would make it possible to eat foods in reasonable portions while still achieving weight loss in a healthy fashion.

At the University of Iowa Hospitals and Clinics in Iowa City, I observed the dietary habits not only of patients, but also of the staff and the visitors to the hospital cafeteria. I noted that in the Eating Disorders Unit, those with anorexia nervosa had a distorted view of what a proper serving of food should be, and, as a result, limited their portion sizes considerably. There was a strong relationship between portion and food selection and physical appearance.

In my previous attempts to lose weight, I had commonly used the measurement units of ¼ cup, ½ cup, ¾ cup, and 1 cup to estimate my portion sizes. I then considered the possibility of basing what I would eat in a day simply on food volume, as determined by cup (8 fluid ounces ≈ 240ml) increments. This concept became the basis for **the CUPS diet®**. And it worked!

Thus, as you can see, the creation and development of **the CUPS diet®** was not only due to my personal desire to lose weight, but also a direct result of my training, experience and knowledge as a physician and psychiatrist.

The Latin word *obesus* describes a condition related to the behavior of overeating, where one has "eaten himself stout, plump, or fat." It is here that my experience as a psychiatrist helped immensely in addressing weight loss. To lose weight, behavior itself must be addressed and controlled.

Today we are less likely to perceive excess weight or obesity merely as a cosmetic problem. There is increasing public awareness of the numerous health associated problems, emotional issues, and psychosocial consequences often caused by this condition. On many occasions my patients discussed the problems that centered around their burden of excess weight: low energy, decreased motivation, and poor self-image.

This lack of energy and decreased motivation causes difficulties at home, school, work and at leisure. At home, individuals tend to participate less frequently in social activities and in developing satisfying personal relationships, which further drives poor self-esteem. At work, low energy and reduced motivation can produce a downward spiral of underperformance that often leads to poor evaluations and eventually a derailed career. Many of my patients also described binge or emotional eating, which, while it may produce feelings of satisfaction in the short-term, almost invariably leads to further weight gain and problems with mood symptoms, such as depression and anxiety.

During my development of **the CUPS diet®** it became clear to me that one of the major hurdles any weight loss plan must overcome results from the fact that many people, while they genuinely desire to lose weight, are unable to commit to a diet. I concluded that the most prevalent reason was that most dieters simply do not want to drastically change foods they have been eating and enjoying in order to comply with the food restrictions found in many of the popular diet plans available today.

My research also showed that many of the popular diets either restrict or limit foods by counting, sorting, weighing or calculating a wide of assortment of different variables such as calories, fat grams, carbohydrates, and the like. Many of the diet books I reviewed were based on limiting calories or food intake by specifying what could and could not be eaten. Also, a significant number of such diets specialized in selling pre-packaged meals, which, for the most part, are not appetizing and are usually rather expensive. **the CUPS diet**® is different.

The unique approach of **the CUPS diet**® to losing weight is scientifically based. It is an ideal tool for sustained and healthy weight loss and yields many benefits. Remember the list of flaws of previous weight loss plans at the start of this chapter? **the CUPS diet**® has been specifically developed without the flaws seen in many other diets. As a result **the CUPS diet**® has numerous advantages over other weight loss methods thus making it a very attractive option for those wanting to lose weight.

the CUPS diet® .....
..... is very easy to start and use
..... is a healthy approach in losing weight
..... considers psychological aspects
..... does not require costly foods
..... does not require supplements
..... lets you enjoy your favorite foods
..... allows for easy meal planning
..... is family-friendly
..... easily allows for dining out
..... uses simple estimating of food intake
..... is very easy to follow in the long-term

This new approach to losing weight is hopefully just what you have been looking for. However, remember that there is no magical road to weight loss. There are only tools to help manage weight. **the CUPS diet**® is one of the most effective of those tools. It is up to you to use it and start shaping your life.

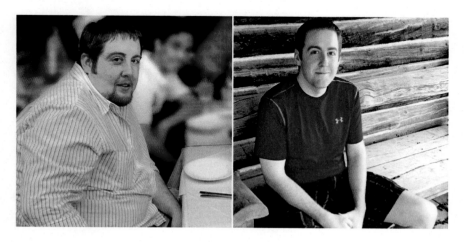

Matt, lost 125 pounds (56.7kg).

He started at 285 pounds (129.3kg) and

was able to get down to a weight of 160 pounds (72.5kg).

Below is his SUCCESS STORY (page 5)

A GREAT DIET

"This has been a great diet for me ... With it (**the CUPS diet**®) I can actually go out and eat and enjoy the foods I love from time to time and still continue to lose weight. Combined with my workout program I have lost more weight and I have been able to keep it off more successfully than I ever had in the past."

CHAPTER TWO

OBESITY – A CHRONIC DISEASE

"Obesity is a chronic disease in the same sense as hypertension and atherosclerosis ..... The excess energy is stored in fat cells that enlarge and/or increase in number. Enlarged fat cells produce the clinical problems associated with obesity either because of the weight or mass of the extra fat or because of the increased secretion of free fatty acids and numerous peptides from enlarged fat cells. The consequence of these two mechanisms is other diseases, such as diabetes mellitus, gallbladder disease, osteoarthritis, heart disease, and some forms of cancer. The spectrum of medical, social, and psychological disabilities includes a range of medical and behavioral problems."
http://academic.research.microsoft.com/Paper/6628118.aspx

This chronic disease has been around for a long time. The Latin word *obesus* was used by Randle Cotgrave in *A Dictionarie of the French and English Tongues* in 1611. *Obesus* comes from *ob,* meaning, "over", and *esus,* which is the past participle of *edere,* meaning "to eat". Together they describe a condition related to the behavior of overeating where one has "eaten himself stout, plump, or fat."

The progression of obesity is often slow, and develops over a long period of time, as is the case with many chronic diseases. Curing chronic diseases, such as obesity, may be difficult, but controlling and preventing them is where the effort is most warranted and should be focused. This is where **the CUPS diet®'s** Control Using PortionS™ model will prove invaluable (page 82).

Body Mass Index

Today we commonly estimate whether someone is obese by using the Body Mass Index concept. Derived from a mathematical formula, the Body Mass Index was created in 1835 by Belgian mathematician Lambert Adolphe Jacques Quetele. Originally known as the Quetele Index, the Body Mass Index (BMI) takes into account both weight and height, that is, mass (kg) divided by height (m)^2.

The Body Mass Index however does not include consideration of body composition (degree of muscularity). This particular index is most reliable for those individuals 19 to 70 years of age, some exceptions being those individuals who are competitive athletes, body builders, pregnant or breast-feeding, or the chronically ill.

BMI Classification

Weight (Class)	BMI
Underweight	< 18.5
Normal Weight	18.5 – 24.9
Overweight	25.0 - 29.9
Obese I	30.0 – 34.9
Obese II	35.0 – 39.9
Obese III*	40.0 >

III* is referred to as Extreme or Morbid Obesity

Your BMI will be provided and updated at www.thecupsdiet.com as you lose weight. To compute Body Mass Index yourself you can use any of a number of online calculators;
www.nhlbisupport.com/bmi/ or www.webmd.com/diet/calc-bmi-plus

Epidemic Proportions

Obesity has reached epidemic proportions in the United States. The number of individuals that are considered overweight (with a BMI of 25.0 to 29.9) or obese (BMI of 30 and over) has increased rapidly in recent decades. Currently one in every six adults worldwide meets the criteria for obesity (WHO's World Health Statistics 2012 report). This trend has been recognized by government health agencies globally. The obesity epidemic is extremely troublesome with regard to increased weight associated health risks and higher financial outlay by both the dieter and society at large.

"Overweight and obesity has reached epidemic proportions in the U.S. and worldwide." *http://www.examiner.com/article/obesity-is-reaching-epidemic-proportions*

"The prevalence of obesity in the United States has doubled in the past two decades."
www.health.gov/dietaryguidelines/dga2005/document/html/chapter3.html

"An estimated 129.6 million Americans ... are overweight or obese."
www.usgovinfo.about.com/cs/healthmedical/a/hhsobesity.html

"The number of overweight and obese Americans has increased since 1960, a trend that shows no signs of slowing down."
www.obesity.org/resources-for/what-is-obesity.html

"... among the group of individuals with a BMI over 30, their average weight continues to increase."
http://www.cdc.gov/media/releases/2012/t0507_weight_nation.html

Weight Associated Health Risks

Many are now aware that being overweight or obese often leads to very serious health consequences. These health related problems are numerous and include such conditions as diabetes, hypertension, stroke, various types of cancer, heart problems, etc. Knowledge of these facts almost invariably results in a genuine desire to lose weight.

Obesity increases the risk of developing:
Coronary heart disease
Type 2 Diabetes
Cancer – endometrial, breast, and colon
Hypertension (high blood pressure)
Dyslipidemia
Liver Disease and Gallbladder Disease
Respiratory Problems
Sleep Apnea
Osteoarthritis
Gynecological problems
http://www.cdc.gov/healthyweight/effects/index.html

Disease Risks Based on BMI

The table is relative to those with a normal weight and waist circumference (40" or less for men and 35" or less for women). Risks are for Diabetes, Hypertension, and Cardiovascular Disease. With an increased waist circumference these risks are even greater.

BMI and Disease Risks

Weight	BMI	Risk	Increased Waist
Underweight	< 18.5		
Normal	18.5–24.9		
Overweight	25–29.9	Increased	HIGH
Obese I	30-34.9	High	VERY HIGH
Obese II	35–39.9	Very High	VERY HIGH
Obese III	40.0 >	Extra High	EXTREMELY HIGH

From the National Heart Lung and Blood Institute

"**Overweight and obesity are the fifth leading risk for global deaths. At least 2.8 million adults die each year as a result of being overweight or obese. In addition, 44% of the diabetes burden, 23% of the ischaemic heart disease burden and between 7% and 41% of certain cancer burdens are attributable to overweight and obesity.**"
http://www.who.int/mediacentre/factsheets/fs311/en/index.html

"**Relative to normal weight … grades 2 and 3 obesity were associated with significantly higher all-cause mortality.**"
www.ncbi.nlm.nih.gov/pubmed/23280227

We Get What We Pay For

With the obesity epidemic this is true, but with a rather disturbing twist. That is, the bigger we get, the more we pay, and pay, and pay.

"**On average, people who are considered obese pay $1,429 (42 percent) more in health care costs than normal-weight individuals.**"
http://win.niddk.nih.gov/statistics/

"**The University of Alabama at Birmingham's hospital, the nation's fourth largest, has widened doors, replaced wall-mounted toilets with floor models able to hold 250 pounds or more, and bought plus size wheelchairs (twice the price of regulars) as well as mini-cranes to hoist obese patients out of bed.**"
www.reuters.com/article/2012/04/30/us-obesity-idUSBRE83T0C820120430

"**The medical care costs of obesity in the United States are staggering. In 2008 dollars, these costs totaled about $147 billion.**"
www.cdc.gov/VitalSigns/AdultObesity

CHAPTER THREE

THE IDEAL WEIGHT

> **Special Note**
>
> *Before starting* **the CUPS diet®** *it is very important that you assess your current* <u>weight associated health risks</u> *(page 33) and also carefully consider your weight loss goals and expectations. Be sure to consult with your doctor to determine whether the state of your health warrants altering your dietary habits by reducing your caloric intake. Seek advice from your doctor as to whether you can safely increase your level of* <u>physical activity</u> *(page 89) to help achieve your weight loss goals.*

When setting about to lose weight, there are three questions you should ask;

1. How much do I WANT to lose?
2. How much do I NEED to lose?
3. How will I stay motivated?

The "How much do I WANT to lose?" question helps define your *"Desired Weight"*. The "How much do I NEED to lose?" question focuses on either the FEAR (<u>health related consequence</u>) or the VANITY (appearance/comfort) related component. And finally, the "How will I stay motivated?" question addresses those techniques that will help keep you committed to your weight loss plan.

When we talk about ideal, normal, healthy, and desired weight, this is what we mean:

Ideal Weight

The notion of an *"Ideal Weight"* is very subjective and can be thought of as a combination of the WANT and NEED questions. It is influenced by many factors, including opinions, preferences, attitudes, and emotions. Objective factors (weight associated health risks, BMI, fat content, etc.) influence this *"Ideal Weight"*, which can be thought of as that which is best overall for **YOU**. In theory it should also be a "Healthy Weight" and will more than likely fall in the normal range of the BMI (page 31).

Normal Weight

Those with a BMI between 18.5 and 24.9 are considered to be within the *"Normal Weight"* range. Because this *"Normal Weight"* is discussed in the context of the BMI it should be noted that it does not take into account a person's body composition (degree of muscularity). This index is most reliable if you are between 19 and 70 years of age, some exceptions being those individuals who are competitive athletes, body builders, pregnant or breast-feeding, or the chronically ill.

Healthy Weight

Today we talk more often about a *"Healthy Weight"* than we do about a *"Normal Weight"*. A *"Healthy Weight"* itself is dependent upon many objective factors as well as your particular body type, which includes your height and waist circumference. *"Healthy Weight"* also addresses the weight associated health risks (page 33) as determined by Body Mass Index.

Desired Weight

"*Desired Weight*" should be thought of as your weight loss goal. This will be asked for when you access the companion website, www.thecupsdiet.com, as directed in CHAPTER SIX. This is the weight that you would be most comfortable with, which would have the lowest weight associated health risks, and would result in looking and feeling your best. It is YOUR "ideal". It is your goal.

Motivation

In order to achieve your weight loss goal, motivation also must be addressed. Motivation is best if it is VERY specific. My experience with users of **the CUPS diet®** reveals that those with the greatest success have motivating factors usually based on either health or appearance. If your primary motivation is health based then be VERY specific. Sometimes it is not enough to simply say; "I want to be healthy." You need to select one VERY specific health related consequence that will keep you motivated. However the level of FEAR of the consequence must be justified and be preventable. Examples of specific FEARS are dying from a heart attack, fear of being paralyzed after having a stroke, or fear of amputation due to diabetic complications, etc... FEAR in itself can be a very powerful motivator.

If motivation is appearance, that is, VANITY driven, then again be VERY specific. It is not enough to say that "I want to look better". One of our SUCCESS STORIES wanted to lose weight 25 pounds for his 50th wedding anniversary and be able to wear the suit he was married in. He did and more. He lost 39 pounds. See SUCCESS STORIES (page 6). These concepts are not mutually exclusive, as a combination of FEAR and VANITY can be very, very, effective.

To keep motivated, use "Success Points". These are steps along the way that will help demonstrate that you are making progress toward reaching your goal. They will vary depending on your BMI (page 31), current weight and your weight loss goal.

The National Institutes of Health (NIH) reports that a reduction of 5-10% of your current body weight will lower your risk for heart disease and other health related conditions. For most people this level of weight loss will be beneficial. This is a very reasonable and realistic goal.

Therefore, one of the most important of the "Success Points" is that of being able to lose 10% of your current body weight with **the CUPS diet®**. After you have lost 10% of your current weight, then set another 10% weight loss goal based on this new weight, and so on, until you are pleased with your weight.

"Success Points"

1. Lower Body Mass Index (BMI)
2. Reaching a new 10 pound (5kg) weight interval
3. Improved weight status category
4. Lower associated health risks (page 33)

↝ Old Chinese Proverb

"It is better to take many small steps in the right direction than to make a great leap forward only to stumble backward."

CHAPTER FOUR

FUNCTIONAL vs. FAD DIETS

the CUPS diet® is a practical weight loss program for those who are obese, those just wanting to lose a few pounds, or those who desire to maintain weight. **the CUPS diet®** can be considered a "functional diet". Functional diets assist in losing weight at a healthy and safe rate, while providing specific and overall health benefits from certain foods or food groups. Weight maintenance can be safely accomplished with this kind of diet as there is no reliance on restricting intake of specific foods or groups. Such restrictions can affect health negatively due to nutritional deficiencies they tend to cause.

Functional diets help broaden your food choices. This is generally accomplished by incorporating healthy alternatives such as vegetables, fresh fruits, natural, and unprocessed foods into meals. On the other hand fad diets tend to restrict, limit, or unrealistically encourage the intake of certain foods or food groups, often through strange or unusual weight loss methods and eating patterns.

Fad diets promote short-term weight loss. Maintenance of that reduced weight is often forfeited. **the CUPS diet®** is quite different, as it can be used to maintain weight loss without compromising health or the satisfaction that comes with eating your favorite foods.

The word "diet" itself can often have a very negative connotation and most of us tend to think of it simply as a way to lose weight.

However, "diet" can mean so much more.

a: food and drink regularly provided or consumed
b: habitual nourishment
c: the kind and amount of food prescribed ... for a special reason
d: a regimen of eating and drinking sparingly so as to reduce one's weight
http://www.merriam-webster.com/dictionary/diet

The last definition is the only one that does not define **the CUPS diet**®. Even though it uses a system of monitoring intake, it does not promote a regimen of eating sparingly to lose weight.

In many ways **the CUPS diet**® is not a diet at all, but rather a new approach to losing weight and maintaining that weight loss. This plan allows for a very practical and simple way to monitor food intake, by its food volume. Its function is to assist in losing weight consistently and at a healthy rate by providing sound nutritional recommendations.

This new type of weight loss and maintenance method is not at all radical or extreme in its approach, as is the case with many fad diets. What you eat now while using **the CUPS diet**® can be the same as after weight has been lost. With only one change, your portions will reflect what is appropriate for you to maintain your weight. You will feel satisfied with this plan. Hunger and cravings are well managed and you will enjoy what you are eating while losing weight. Awareness of how much food is appropriate increases as you use **the CUPS diet**®.

The actual amount of weight lost is influenced by many factors:

* Metabolic factors (page 85)
* Food types eaten
* Genetic predisposition
* Physical activity levels (page 89)

In its approach to losing weight, **the CUPS diet**® is unique, as you can eat any of your favorite foods while simply controlling how much you eat in an average day. This is accomplished by monitoring food intake with the use of measuring cup (8 fl. oz. ≈ 240ml) based increments (¼ cup, ½ cup, ¾ cup, 1 cup, etc.). **the CUPS diet**® is not about eating a cup of this or a cup of that. You decide how many cups to eat at each meal or snack. These cup based increments are used only to track food intake.

the CUPS diet® provides a very easy way to control how much food is right for you.

Enjoy life.

Eat what you want.

You're in control.

IT'S SIMPLE.

CHAPTER FIVE

HOW the CUPS diet® WORKS

the CUPS diet® is based upon three principles:

Control Using PortionS™
Basal Metabolic Rate - **BMR**
Adjusted Individual Measurement – **AIM** (page 44)

Control Using PortionS™

The method of weight management (losing, gaining, or maintaining) that is based upon the use of measuring cup (8 fl. oz. ≈ 240ml) increments is Control Using PortionS™. This is the foundation for the great success of **the CUPS diet®**, see SUCCESS STORIES (page 5).

Weight loss ultimately results from using more calories (energy), than consumed. To lose one lb. (0.45kg), about 3,500 calories must be burnt. To lose this pound within a week, one needs to control and reduce food consumption so it amounts to an average of a 500 calorie deficit every day. The alternative is to increase activity in order to use these 3,500 calories over the course of a week. The combination of modifying food intake (dieting) while increasing physical activity (exercising) is the best overall approach to losing weight at a healthy and consistent rate.

Portion vs. Serving

So, what is a portion? What is a serving?

Portion

A portion is not the same as a serving. Simply put, a portion is how much you choose to eat, and a serving is a recommended or standard amount of a food, usually based upon nutritional guidelines. A serving may be more or less than a particular portion of a food or beverage you may have chosen.

While following the **CUPS diet®** you will not be required to eat a cup of this or a cup of that, and you will not have to eat your food out of cups. Measuring cup increments are used only as a way to track your daily food intake, your AIM (page 44).

Basal Metabolic Rate

The scientifically based concept at the foundation of **the CUPS diet®** is the resting Basal Metabolic Rate. It helps to determine the amount of food that can be eaten on a daily basis. This recommended amount of food is called the Adjusted Individual Measurement – **AIM**. It helps achieve optimum weight loss and successfully maintain your program of weight management (losing, gaining, or maintaining weight).

Basal Metabolic Rate represents the minimum calories necessary to sustain many bodily functions such as respiration, cardiovascular systemics, and maintenance of body temperature. It is lowest at rest after sleep and after a 12-hour fast. It accounts for about 60% of total daily energy expenditure and is the greatest single component used in determining the "daily" resting metabolic rate.

A number of factors influence your BMR. Many interact with each other. Some of these can be controlled and some are natural processes which we can do little to alter. However, by following **the CUPS diet**® and its guidelines for consistent weight loss, you will help keep your Basal Metabolic Rate at a level that will promote that weight loss.

BMR can be determined by using a number of different mathematical formulas and procedures. The formula that is used by **the CUPS diet**® is the Revised Harris-Benedict Equation.

*SPECIAL NOTE: When using **the CUPS diet**® it will never be necessary for you to calculate your own BMR, as this will be done for you automatically with every update in your weight, at the companion website and used to help determine your own personal **AIM**.

Adjusted Individual Measurement

AIM is the volume of food, quantified in measuring cup increments, which you should use as a target regarding food consumption to ensure consistent and healthy weight loss. It should be thought of as the most you should eat in day. You do not have to eat your **AIM** amount every day. If you feel full then it is perfectly fine to stop eating.

Remember that this is only your target so that you will not overeat. It should be noted that individuals who consume 100% of their **AIM** on a daily basis consistently lose weight 90% of the time, whereas those that eat up to 90% of their **AIM** lose weight nearly 100% of the time.

Here is one place in life where coming close to your target is actually better than hitting it. In CHAPTER SIX, **How much can I eat?**, details are provided on obtaining your AIM (steps, 1-8).

Companion Website

CHAPTER SIX

HOW MUCH CAN I EAT?

Adjusted Individual Measurement (AIM)

One of the most important aspects of **the CUPS diet®** is the concept of the **AIM** (page 44). This is what you are "aiming" at in eating in a typical day in measuring cup increments. Below are details on how to obtain your **AIM**.

Obtaining your AIM
1. Visit www.thecupsdiet.com
2. On the home page select the Book Access tab
3. Enter the access information and select Sign Up
4. Enter your email and password and then Sign In
5. Select Update Weekly Weight
6. Enter your weight (lbs.)
7. Then select Update Weight
8. Your AIM will be shown on the left

A special conversion factor is used in conjunction with the Basal Metabolic Rate to arrive at your **AIM** (page 44). The formula for its calculation has been programmed within the website so that you do not need to perform any calculations. By focusing on the BMR (page 43) you can be assured that while dieting you will have an appropriate amount of food to eat in an average day so that you will not be hungry or dissatisfied with your meal choices.

Adjusted – adjusted with weight updates
Individual – based upon your own BMR
Measurement – measuring cup increments

The concept of the **AIM** (page 44) allows this diet program to be truly individualized for each person and have ranged from 5 to 13 cups a day for those that have used **the CUPS diet**®. Examples of actual user's **AIM** amounts follow below:

Age and Gender	Weight	AIM
32 year old male	281 (127kg)	**10**
55 year old male	310 (140kg)	**9.5**
43 year old female	190 (86kg)	**6.5**
48 year old female	180 (81kg)	**6**

AIM is an easy way to keep track of your food intake, especially with the My Daily Progress tracking calendar, discussed in CHAPTER SEVEN (page 49). It is your target indicating how much to eat to ensure consistent and healthy weight loss. You do not have to eat your **AIM** every day of the week. If you feel full and have eaten less than your **AIM**, then it is fine to stop eating. The key lies in averaging your food intake over the week. Routinely having 2 cups below your current **AIM** is not recommended.

Your **AIM** will be recalculated every week as you Update Weekly Weight and it will decrease slowly in ½ cup increments as you lose weight. This is because as you experience weight loss, your body will require fewer calories. If, after 2 consecutive weeks there is no change in weight, **AIM** will be reduced by ½ cup, and if you gain weight in a week, it will be reduced by ½ cup. These changes are needed to compensate for the dreaded "stall-out" that some are prone to.

To break "plateaus" where your weight loss has stalled, try changing your eating habits. For example if your **AIM** was 7 and intake has been a fairly consistent 7 cups every day, try having one or two splurge days, and reduce your intake accordingly on the other days of the week, all the while continuing to average 7 cups a day for the week. Also add more physical activity to your daily routine.

Do not become discouraged if weight loss does not begin immediately. Because of the wide variation in factors affecting BMR (page 43) and the proficiency of individuals in estimating cup amounts, **AIM** (page 44) adjustments may be warranted so as to optimize your weight loss efforts.

In **the CUPS diet®** no compensation has been made for exercise as it relates to food intake. Some programs allow you to have a more to eat when you exercise, however, the goal of **the CUPS diet®** has been to focus on consistent weight loss for the long run and encourage exercise in order to maintain that loss.

the CUPS diet®'s #1 loser (page 5), who lost 125 lbs. (56.7kg), became very involved in working out regularly at the gym as well as training in Kempo Karate. I worked very closely with him and encouraged him to continue to stick to his **AIM** regardless of the intensity of his workouts. And .... it worked, as he lost weight and increased his strength and endurance.

YOUR GOAL should be to stay within your **AIM**. Workouts will promote lean tissue growth and will promote a higher **metabolism** and thus weight loss. Your own **AIM** should be sufficient in providing the **necessary nutrients needed** with a program of regular physical activity (page 89).

CHAPTER SEVEN

USING the CUPS diet®

RECIPE for WEIGHT LOSS

SERVES: the Entire Family
SPECIAL INGREDIENTS: None
LEVEL of DIFFICULTY: Very Easy
RATING: ★★★★★

INGREDIENTS:
eReader/Computer/Tablet/Smartphone
Companion Website Access
the CUPS diet® book by Dr. Mascaro
AIM (**A**djusted **I**ndividual **M**easurement)
3 Meals Every Day
2 Snacks Throughout the Day
5 or More Glasses of Water Daily

Plus .... a generous portion of "Belief"

Directions for Daily Use

After setting up your website access, obtaining your **AIM** (page 46), reviewing your Wt. Associated Health Risks, and finishing your book, you can start using **the CUPS diet®**. *** If you have set up your FREE account skip steps 2-3.**

Using the CUPS diet®

1. Visit www.thecupsdiet.com
2. *** On the home page select the blue** Book Access **tab**
3. *** Enter the access information requested**
4. Select my account (upper right corner)
5. Enter your email and password and then Sign In
6a. Select NEW USERS START HERE or
6b. Then select Update Weekly Weight
7. Enter weight (lbs.) and **Update Weight**
8a. Select **Continue** and the day of the week
.... enter your cups eaten and then Save or
8b. Select Record Your CUPS
.... enter your cups eaten and then Save
9. You can now view My Daily Progress

It is best to start **the CUPS diet®** and subsequently Update Weekly Weight at the beginning of the week. Sunday is the best day to use as a "start day" as it matches well with the progress tracking calendar, at the My Daily Progress tab. However, you can use different days to update your weekly weight.

One benefit of choosing Sunday as a "start day" is that it serves as a reminder that even if you do go over your **AIM** (page 44), averaged for the week, you can start over again on the following Sunday. There is always another Sunday, always another "new" day, and always another "new" week. Also, as the weekend nears, you may be able to exhibit a little more self-control over any possible over-indulgences on Friday or Saturday night, especially when you know you will have to step on the scale Sunday morning and Update Weekly Weight.

Digital scales, which are optional, usually show weight to the nearest two tenths of a pound and will help track your weight loss progress more effectively. Simply step on the scale in the morning of your start day (before you eat or drink anything) and until you get the same reading twice. Use that as your starting weight for the week. There is no reason to step back on the scale until the next "beginning of the week" day.

In fact, weighing yourself more than once a week is discouraged as weight can fluctuate by up to 5 lbs. (2.2kg) within a 24-hour period due to food or fluid intake and changes in activity level. As long as you adhere to **the CUPS diet®** recommendations, any ups and downs in weight will be averaged out, with the overall trend downward. Your weight associated health risks are updated with changes in your weekly weight (as it affects your BMI).

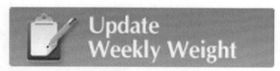

*Screenshot "**Update Weekly Weight**" tab and text from the companion website, https://www.thecupsdiet.com/index.cfm*

Enter your Sunday morning weight. "Update Weight" will update your Health Risk factors, BMI, and AIM. "Continue" will take you to My Daily Progress where you can Record Your CUPS or review your progress.

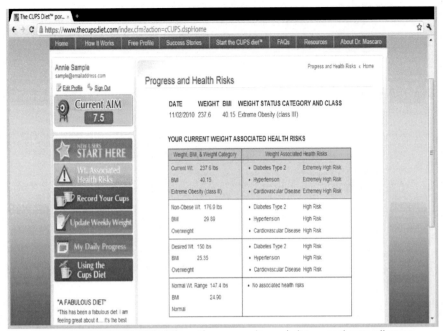

*Screenshot "**HEALTH RISKS**" from the companion website, www.thecupsdiet.com*

Your **AIM** (page 44) may change every few weeks with changes in your BMR. Along the left side of all user webpages you will note the user color coded tabs - NEW USERS START HERE, Wt. Associated Health Risks, Record Your CUPS, Update Weekly Weight, My Daily Progress and Using the CUPS diet with details on how to use the diet for those not using the book.

The green tab, My Daily Progress, or the blue tab, Record Your CUPS, allows you to record your food and water (in cups) for any day of the week. For best results enter cups by the meal rather than the day. You can, however, combine entry styles throughout the week.

Record Your CUPS for Monday, November 1, 2010

Enter your CUPS eaten below. By selecting "Save" you will update your CUPS for the day in "My Daily Progress" based upon your last entry. You may enter CUPS for meals throughout the day or at the end of the day or simply the total amount for the day. Combination of both types of tracking methods within the week is also permissible. Meal tracking however, is recommended for the best weight loss.

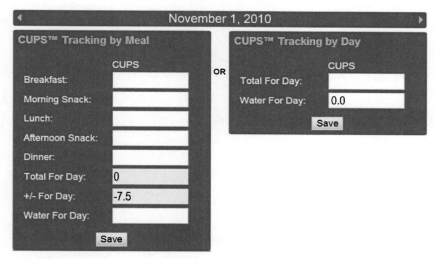

*Screenshot "**RECORD YOUR CUPS**" from the companion website, www.thecupsdiet.com*

the CUPS diet® allows YOU to decide how much YOU want to eat at meals. It is best to have at least 1 cup per meal, and at least ½ cup for each snack. This ½ - 1 cup recommendation for meals or snacks is independent of whether or not it counts toward your AIM. For example, you may have ½ cup of fresh fruit for a snack, which equals ½ cup. However if this is one of your first 2 cups of fresh fruit in that day, you do not have to count it toward your AIM. For optimum results, keep track of your food intake for each of your 5 daily meals (3 meals and 2 snacks) as the day progresses and record your cups. Try to have an 8 oz. (240ml) glass of water at each meal and snack and record your water intake for the day.

NOTE: You can return at any time and sign in at my account in the upper right of the homepage.

Using the companion website makes it very easy to keep track of your food intake. By selecting My Daily Progress you can see how you are doing for the day in regard to your **AIM** (page 44) and how you are doing for the week or month as well as selecting the day of the month to enter or make changes in food intake.

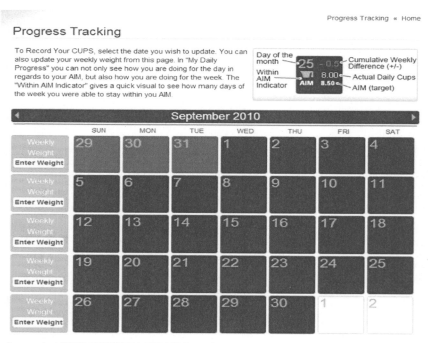

*Screenshot "**PROGRESS TRACKING**" from the companion website, www.thecupsdiet.com*

The "Within **AIM** Indicator" gives you a quick visual to see how many days of the week you were able to stay within your **AIM** and how you are doing for the week, that is, if you are under (-) or over (+) your **AIM** for the week. The cumulative weekly difference colors, **Green (-/under)** and Red (+/over) represent the cumulative difference in your **AIM** (page 44) for the week and will reset at the start of each week.

Progress Tracking

To Record Your CUPS, select the date you wish to update. You can also update your weekly weight from this page. In "My Daily Progress" you can not only see how you are doing for the day in regards to your AIM, but also how you are doing for the week. The "Within AIM Indicator" gives a quick visual to see how many days of the week you were able to stay within you AIM.

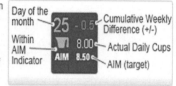

*Screenshot "**PROGRESS TRACKING SYMBOLS**" from the companion website, www.thecupsdiet.com*

The "Actual User's Progress Tracking" that is shown next helps illustrate how flexible **the CUPS diet®** can really be. You do not need to eat the same amount every day. For example, if your **AIM** were 7, then for the week you should not go over 49 cups. You can split up these 49 cups throughout the week based upon your needs and lifestyle.

If you have a special "event" such as a birthday party or a dinner function and you know it will be difficult to stay within your **AIM**, and then plan ahead. For two days before and two days after the "event", reduce your food intake by up to 2 cups for each of these four days. Then when the day of your "event" you can take these cups not eaten in these four days, that is 8 cups, and add them to your **AIM** of 7 cups for a total or 15 cups available at your dinner function, party, etc.

	SUN	MON	TUE	WED	THU	FRI	SAT
Weekly Weight 427.9	28 −1.00 0.00 AIM 10.5	1 −1.00 9.50 AIM 10.5	2 −2.50 9.00 AIM 10.5	3 −3.50 9.50 AIM 10.5	4 −4.00 10.00 AIM 10.0	5 −4.50 10.00 AIM 10.5	6 −6.00 9.00 AIM 10.5
Weekly Weight 414.9	7 −2.00 8.00 AIM 10.0	8 −1.50 10.50 AIM 10.0	9 −3.50 8.00 AIM 10.0	10 −7.50 6.00 AIM 10.0	11 −8.50 9.00 AIM 10.0	12 −8.50 10.00 AIM 10.0	13 0.00 AIM 10.0
Weekly Weight 413.8	14 −1.00 9.00 AIM 10.0	15 −6.00 3.00 AIM 10.0	16 −8.00 10.00 AIM 10.0	17 −8.00 10.00 AIM 10.0	18 −10.50 7.50 AIM 10.0	19 −9.50 11.00 AIM 10.0	20 −11.50 8.00 AIM 10.0
Weekly Weight 412.2	21 −3.00 7.00 AIM 10.0	22 −5.50 7.50 AIM 10.0	23 −6.50 9.00 AIM 10.0	24 −7.50 9.00 AIM 10.0	25 −6.00 11.50 AIM 10.0	26 −4.00 12.00 AIM 10.0	27 −2.00 12.00 AIM 10.0

Screenshot "ACTUAL USER'S PROGRESS TRACKING" from the companion website, www.thecupsdiet.com

Once you have achieved your goal, increase your **AIM** by ½ cup every week until you see that you are starting to gain weight and then reduce your **AIM** by ½ cup thereafter. You may have to from time to time make adjustments in your **AIM** (page 44) to the point where you will be able to maintain your ideal weight.

Remember to update your weight weekly. When you sign in you can go directly to Record Your CUPS and enter your intake. Review CHAPTERS EIGHT-TWELVE to learn more about estimating portions.

Appendix II contains sample meals and Appendix III contains a listing of Food Approximation in CUPS (page 117).

CHAPTER EIGHT

ESTIMATING PORTIONS

Estimating Food Volume

Below are some common items along with their "CUP" equivalent. This can be of assistance in helping to estimate food volume and portion size:

¼ CUP
Egg, Golf Ball, Pager, Finger, or a Bite of Food
½ CUP
Slice of Bread, Deck of Cards, or a Cell Phone
¾ CUP
6 fluid ounce Wine Glass (180ml), Three Fingers, or a Tennis Ball
1 CUP
8 fluid ounce Carton of Milk (240ml), or a Baseball
1½ CUPS
12 fluid ounce (360ml) Soda Can, Coffee Mug, or an Average Fist

When using **the CUPS diet®** it is not necessary to measure everything you eat, as many foods will count a certain amount regardless of their particular size. Estimating cup amounts is all about imagining how much volume a portion of food will occupy, such as eggs, for example. As previously noted, an egg will count as ¼ cup regardless of its size (small, medium, large, extra-large, or jumbo). This helps simplify the estimating of cups amounts.

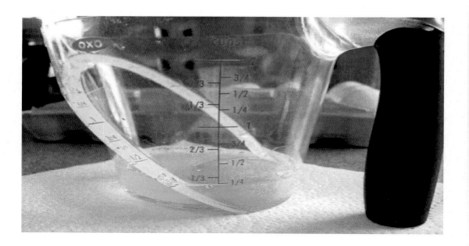

Common containers can be utilized to represent the volume of 1 cup, ¾ cup, ½ cup, or even ¼ cup of food. This is very useful in estimating portion sizes. You will also find that odd sized containers (rectangular, square, round or even oblong) can be easily converted into their cup equivalent visually.

Even though estimating portions is determined with measuring cup (8 fl. oz. ≈ 240ml) based increments, you NEVER need to carry measuring cups or any other cumbersome implements with you. You will be amazed how quickly you will get the knack of visualizing and being able to estimate the volume of what you eat. Measuring cups themselves can also be very handy at home, especially when starting **the CUPS diet®**.

Always round up any estimation of cups to the next highest ¼ cup increment. In other words, if you are not sure whether to count a portion as a ¼ cup or a ½ cup, then it should be counted as ½ cup. Not all bites of food will equal a ¼ cup, however if you have only one bite of a single type of food, then, because it is necessary to round to the next highest cup increment.

Try to estimate the volume (your cups amount) of a portion of food realistically. Remember, no smashing of your food before estimating its cup equivalent. If the food or the portion you are eating is too large to approximate easily, then you should probably ask whether it is appropriate to be eating a smaller amount in the first place.

It is usually much easier to estimate smaller portions of food than larger portions. This too may help give you motivation to eat smaller portions of food and thus lose weight more consistently.

Estimating LARGE Portions

If the portion of food is larger than your fist, imagine cutting it in half and then estimate that half's cup amount and is that times two for the entire portion.

A very easy and optional way of estimating any large portion of food is to use your own hand as a measuring device to calculate the amount of "CUPS" in a particular portion. First you will have to estimate the size of your own hand. This can be achieved by conducting a very simple in-house kitchen procedure.

	Estimating LARGE Portions
1	You will need two separate containers
	..... your fist should be able to easily fit into the 1st container
2	Place the 1st container into the 2nd container
3	Fill the 1st container completely full of water
4	Now insert your fist into the 1st container up to your wrist
5	Measure the water that has spilled out of the 1st container
	..... use measuring cup amounts for this measurement
6	This amount (1 – 1½ cups) is what your hand or fist would represent

This estimation/visualizing technique makes it easy when dining out to estimate the food you are eating. This is true especially in the case of irregularly shaped portions (pizza, sandwiches, mashed potatoes, fast foods, and scoops of anything) or large portions.

Eventually, as you become more familiar with **the CUPS diet®**, you will find you can easily visualize what you are eating and estimate how many CUPS it represent.

Next you will find measurement equivalent tables to help estimate your CUPS amount. Keep in mind that you never have to actually weigh or measure your portions. These "equivalents" are only here to assist your estimating of food portions when you know their weight, volume, or diameter.

Equivalents

CUPS	fl. oz.	ml	tbsp.	tsp.
	0.16	5ml	0.33	1
	½	15ml	1	3
	1	30ml	2	6
¼	2	60ml	4	12
½	4	120ml	8	24
¾	6	180ml	12	36
1	8	240ml	16	48
1¼	10	300ml	20	60
1½	12	360ml	24	72

ounce	pound	gram	kilogram
1		28g	
2		56g	
3		85g	
4	0.25	113g	0.11kg
8	0.50	226g	0.22kg
12	0.75	340g	0.34kg
16	1	453g	0.45kg

inch	centimeter
1	2.5 cm
2	5.1 cm
3	7.6 cm
4	10.2 cm
5	12.7 cm

CUPS Approximation Examples (photo)

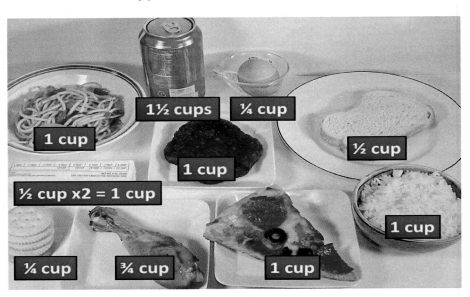

Food	Portion	CUPS
Crackers	5 round crackers	¼
Egg	1 whole egg	¼
Beef	¼ lb. is 4 oz. (113g)	1
Bread	1 average slice of bread	½
Butter [**Cx2**]	1 stick or ½ cup is 4 oz.	½ **x2** = 1
Chicken	3 oz. (85g) leg – grilled	¾
Pasta	1 cup (cooked)	1
Pizza	small slice of pizza	1
Rice	1 cup (cooked)	1
Soda	1½ cup is 12 fl. oz.	1½

CHAPTER NINE

FOOD GROUPS and CATEGORIES

There are five FOOD GROUPS and five SPECIAL FOOD CATEGORIES in **the CUPS diet**®. A FOOD GROUP helps to classify foods while a SPECIAL FOOD CATEGORY assists in determining cup calculations. SPECIAL FOOD CATEGORIES may also include different FOOD GROUPS.

FOOD GROUPS

	The Five Food Groups
1	Vegetables
2	Fruits – does not include juices (page 64)
3	Dairy Products (page 64)
4	Grains and Breads (page 64)
5	Meats – includes poultry and seafood (page 65)

1. Vegetables

Most vegetables (including salads) will not count toward your **AIM** when they consist only of vegetables that are NOT part of the SPECIAL FOOD CATEGORY, the **CUP** for **CUP** vegetables [**C/C**]. Try to have at least 2 cups of vegetables every day with your meals and choose a variety of different types (**COUPLE** of **CUPS** recommendation in CHAPTER TWELVE). Toppings (salad dressings, cheeses, meats, fruits, and croutons, etc.) may count. Any salad that has salad dressing on it will count at least ¼ cup and usually ½ cup. For items that might be added to a salad, estimate them as if they were being eaten separately. See CHAPTER ELEVEN,

"CONDIMENTS" for details on special food recommendations that may apply to toppings for vegetables or salads.

2. Fruits

Include fruit at every meal (fresh if possible) and in snacks. Frozen fruit, canned fruit, and fruit juices always count toward your AIM (page 44). Some fruits (apples, bananas, oranges, etc.), count as one cup, regardless of size. Fresh Fruits are included in a SPECIAL FOOD CATEGORY, First Fruits Free [FFF]. Fruit provides fiber, which is instrumental in slowing the digestive process. They will help you feel satisfied, despite the fact that they are low in fats and calories and can be an important factor in helping you lose weight.

3. Dairy Products

A variety of dairy products (milk, yogurt, cheese, and eggs) should be included in your meals when using **the CUPS diet®**, with an emphasis on fat free or low fat dairy products if possible. Some dairy products are included in the SPECIAL FOOD CATEGORY of the Count times 2 [Cx2] foods. Calcium contained in dairy products plays a very positive role in weight loss. Dairy products are a good source of protein, vitamins A and D and phosphorus.

4. Grains

When possible, try to eat whole grain foods. And once again, vary your food selections. Some grains (breads, cereal, rice, crackers, and pasta) are also found in the SPECIAL FOOD CATEGORY of the Count times 2 [Cx2] foods. Grains are an excellent source of protein and dietary fiber, which is instrumental in slowing the digestive process. Whole grains are found in whole wheat flour, whole wheat bread, oatmeal, grits, corn tortillas, and brown rice.

5. Meats

This FOOD GROUP is a major source of protein. Foods in this group also contain iron, vitamin B12 and zinc. Meat consumption is not required and vegetarians or vegans can easily prescribe to these diet guidelines. Substitutes for meats, such as beans, tofu, lentils, and chickpeas will help provide protein. See SPECIAL FOOD CATEGORY on "**M**eat" [**M**] for more details (page 68).

SPECIAL FOOD CATEGORIES

SPECIAL FOOD CATEGORIES consist of foods that have unique criteria for determining their cup amounts.

Special Food Category Reminders	
Cx2	**Count times 2** – foods are counted twice
C/C	**C** for **CUP** vegetables – always count towards your **AIM** (page 44)
U	
P	
FFF	**First Fruits Free** – two fresh fruits in a day do not count (page 67)
M	**Meats** – lean pref., 4 oz. (113g) **counts (CTS)** as 1 cup (page 68)
Ø	**NO** count foods and beverages (page 69)

1. Count times 2 [Cx2]

is a special category of foods that, because of their nutritional composition, are counted twice when determining intake. For these foods all cup amounts must be doubled. As a result most foods in this category will count at least ½ cup.

For example, 1 oz. of cheese counts as ¼ cup, but it must be counted twice as it is a **Cx2** food, so that it ultimately will be counted as ½ cup. As an aid in remembering specific foods in this category, recall that **C**ount begins with the letter "C" and that many of the foods in this category can be recalled as the foods/types which also begin with "**C**".

Not all foods that begin with the letter "C" are counted twice. There are foods that do not begin with "**C**" that are also **Cx2** foods. These foods are similar to their letter "C" counterpart. The cup amounts for the **Cx2** foods are listed within Appendix III.

DAIRY [Cx2] – LFP
Cx2 Cheese - all types
Cx2 Christmas (Eggnog)
Cx2 Condensed Milk, Evaporated Milk
Cx2 Cream, Ice **C**ream,
Cx2 Butter, Margarine
Cx2 Sour **C**ream, Mayonnaise
Cx2 Crème Brûlée, **C**ustard, Flan
Cx2 DQ Blizzard **C**ookie Dough

DESERTS [Cx2] and SWEETS [Cx2] – LFP
Cx2 Cake, **C**upcake, Pastry, Pie
Cx2 Candy, **C**andy Bar
Cx2 Caramel, **C**hocolate, Fudge
Cx2 Cookies, Brownies, Doughnuts

MISCELLANEOUS [Cx2]
Cx2 Cashews, Nuts (any type)
Cx2 Crisco (shortening), Lard, Oil
Cx2 Crispy, Battered or Fried foods

Cx2 Cornmeal, Flour
Cx2 Sugar - after the 1st tsp. (5ml)

"**From the CUPboard**" contains **Mascaro Family Recipes** (page 162). The total cup amount for each recipe has been listed below the ingredients and has already taken into account any SPECIAL FOOD CATEGORY instructions, such as the **Cx2** foods.

2. CUP for CUP vegetables [C/C]

is a SPECIAL FOOD CATEGORY of vegetables that count as estimated, that is, "cup for cup", when determining intake. All other vegetables do not count toward your **AIM** (page 44). Vegetables that do count include **C** = **C**orn and **C**orn products, **U** = leg**U**mes, which include beans, bean products (except for green beans) as well as lentils, and chickpeas), and **P**= **P**otatoes and **P**otato (page 161) products. To recall these vegetables:

.....**C**orn
leg**U**mes
.....**P**otatoes

3. First Fruits Free [FFF]

Your **F**irst 2 cups in a day of **F**resh **F**ruit (page 67) will not count toward your **AIM**. If not a FRESH fruit then count it cup for cup. Beyond your first 2 cups any fresh fruit will count. Fresh fruits not eaten in a day cannot be carried over to the next day.

the CUPS diet® focuses on enabling you to control portions easily and not become consumed with detailed measuring and weighing. Some fruits (apples, bananas, oranges, etc.), count as one cup, regardless of their size. So if you are going to have an apple, then have it, and have a big one, and enjoy it! After all, it counts the same as a small one. If you have an apple (which counts 1 cup) and a banana (1 cup) and an orange (1 cup), you will only have to count the last cup, that is, toward your AIM (page 44). Choose different fresh fruits if possible. See Food Approximation in CUPS tables in APPENDIX III.

Remember:

First – First 2 cups of fresh fruit in a day
Fruits – Fresh (does not include juices or canned)
Free – Does not count toward your AIM

4. Meats [M]

Is not only a FOOD GROUP, it is also a SPECIAL FOOD CATEGORY because meat approximations can vary to a large degree. The cup approximation for meats has been simplified and is based upon a 4 oz. (113g) portion.

This 4 oz. portion of any meat product (beef, pork, sausage, poultry, or fish, etc.) will always count as the volume of 1 cup (8 fluid ounces ≈240ml) and is for reference purposes only. Utilizing it will eliminate the need to actually weigh foods from this SPECIAL FOOD CATEGORY and will assist you in shopping for food, preparing meals, and determining cup amounts very quickly.

Up to a **COUPLE** of **CUPS** of meat a day is suggested when following **the CUPS diet**®. Meat products, such as bologna or ham, count as ¼ cup for each slice and low fat is recommended. As for foods such as tacos, sandwiches, or gyros, it makes no difference whether you have beef, pork, lamb, or chicken when calculating your cups, as 4 oz. counts (**CTS**) 1 cup, 2 oz. **CTS** ½ cup and 1 oz. **CTS** ¼ cup.

If you were however to have fried, battered, or breaded meat, then that would count twice as it is a **Cx2** food, as noted above where **C** = **C**rispy, battered or fried food.

For example, an average chicken leg might weigh 3 oz. (85g) and if 4 oz. (113g) of meat is 1 cup, then 3 oz. would be equivalent to ¾ cup, but because it is a **Cx2** food, it counts double and thus equals 1½ cups (12 fluid ounces ≈ 360ml).

5. NO count foods & beverages [Ø]

This is a SPECIAL FOOD CATEGORY that includes foods and beverages that do not count toward your **AIM**, unless they are included in the [**FFF**] SPECIAL FOOD CATEGORY (page 67) or they are *coconut water or *juices (tomato, vegetable, or V8) of which your 1st cup in a day does not count toward your **AIM** amount.

BEVERAGES:

    Coffee or Diet Soda or Tea or Water
    *Coconut water
    *Juices - Vegetable or Tomato or V8

FOODS:

    2 Fresh Fruits a day [**FFF**]
    Vegetables, unless a [**C/C**] food (page 67)

MISCELLANEOUS:

Artificial Sweetener, Baking Powder or Soda
Broth, Capers, Herbs, Horseradish, Hot Sauce
Lemon Juice, Lime Juice, Mustard
Pico de Gallo, Pickled Ginger, Salsa
Spices, Vegetable Spreads
Very Very Low Calorie Gelatin
Wasabi, Worcestershire Sauce
the **NO** count Vegetables
tsp. of any Condiment (page 79)

CHAPTER TEN

MEALS, SNACKS, and WATER

Meals

the CUPS diet® allows YOU to decide how much YOU want to eat at each meal (breakfast, lunch and dinner) or snack. Try to eat at least 1 cup (countable or not) per meal, and at least ½ cup (countable or not) for each snack. Try to have your last meal at least three hours before bedtime.

Breakfast

You may have heard your mother say "breakfast is the most important meal of the day." Well, mom was right. Have breakfast within 30 to 60 minutes of getting up. This can help stimulate or "kick start" your metabolism, which helps promote weight loss. Eat ½ to 3 cups depending upon your **AIM**. Vary your breakfast daily, and be sure to include protein, dairy, fruit and grains.

A study was prepared by the Department of Psychology at the University of Texas in El Paso, Texas, and published in The American Society for Nutritional Science in January of 2004. This study was entitled <u>The Time of Day of Food Intake Influences Overall Intake in Humans</u>, *John M. de Castro, Department of Psychology, University of Texas at El Paso, El Paso, TX.* The researchers studied the food diaries of a number of men and women. They found that, of the 867 male and female subjects that were studied, those eating their meals earlier in the day felt more satisfied in the morning, and thus they found it easier to reduce the total amount of food eaten for the entire day.

In 2002, The North American Association for the Study of Obesity published results from a cross-sectional study of 2,959 people in the National Weight Control Registry Conference Report (NWCR). This registry was composed of both men and women who had lost an average of 70 pounds (31.75kg) and had managed to maintain that seventy pound weight loss for more than six years. Seventy eight percent of those individuals were found to have made a practice of eating breakfast regularly every day of the week.

Example of a Breakfast

Next is a 2 cup breakfast example. In APPENDIX II (page 90) there are more examples of meals with nutritional breakdowns. These "examples" illustrate the ease of determining food intake.

Portion	Breakfast	CUPS
cup or more	WATER [0]	0
cup	COFFEE [0] or TEA [0] is optional	0
¼ cup = 25	BLUEBERRIES [FFF] (page 64 and 149)	0
small	BAGEL, up to 3" diameter (page 122)	0.50
2 tbsp. = 1 oz.	+ Cream Cheese [Cx2] is ¼ cup x2	0.50
	FRUIT SMOOTHIE:	
¼ cup = 3 medium	..... Strawberries [FFF]	0
cup	..... Milk – LFP	0.75
1	EGG – scrambled	0.25
½ cup	+ Green Peppers [0]	0

Snacks

Regulated snacking helps control appetite and assists with weight loss. How much you eat will be for the most part dictated by your **AIM** (page 44), and whether or not you have planned any "over the **AIM** days". Eat slowly to give your body time to react to your food, and send a signal to your brain (received up to 20 minutes later) that you are getting full.

Snacks (unless indicated) and any other foods that you use as a snack are always included in your **AIM**. Try to have two different snacks every day and eat the equivalent of at least ½ cup (4 fluid ounces ≈ 120ml) for each snack. Remember to drink one cup of water with your snacks. See APPENDIX III – Snacks, for examples of snacks and how to estimate their cups (page 156).

Water

A study in the Journal of Clinical Endocrinology and Metabolism reported that drinking water increases the metabolic rate. Drinking cold water can assist with boosting metabolism even more. Always consider water a very important part of your weight loss plan.
www.livestrong.com/article/521032-does-drinking-cold-water-help-speed-up-your-metabolism/

Try to drink one cup (8 fluid ounces ≈ 240ml) of water with each meal and snack for a minimum of five cups daily. Schedule your water intake about 15 to 20 minutes before eating your meal or snack. This can increase a feeling of "fullness" which, as a result, will reduce your appetite level. Water also helps to promote the utilization of fat and remove the waste products of fat breakdown.

Many have recommended drinking eight glasses of water a day. I tried that when I was developing **the CUPS diet**®. And it worked! I

lost weight BUT I also lost my social life. I found that all I was doing was going to the bathroom. So over time I cut my water from 8 to 7 to 6 and then to 5. Five glasses of water for me and many others on the diet and seemed to be a good number to work with. It also matched well with eating five times a day, that is, three meals and two snacks. If it works for you to have more than five glasses, that is great. The key is to stay well hydrated, as thirst itself can at times be mistaken for hunger.
(U.S. Public Health Service Commissioned Corps)

Daily Menu "SAMPLE"

Following are a number of sample menus (breakfast, lunch, dinner, snacks) for an entire day. These particular menus total 6½ cups of food intake for an individual with an **A**djusted **I**ndividual **M**easurement of 7 cups. Note that this is only a **"SAMPLE" Daily Menu** to help put into perspective how simple meal planning and cup determination is. These menus are followed by an actual Record Your CUPS screenshot (page 78) with the cups amounts entered in for each meal (breakfast , lunch, dinner) and each snack to illustrate the ease of keeping track of your intake while using **the CUPS diet®**.

For descriptive purposes, tracking by the meal AND by the day have been entered on page 78. Meal tracking is preferred and gives you the best overall results. Note that the **AIM** used in this **"SAMPLE"** is 7 cups, and is ONLY an example. Your **AIM** will be determined from your individual own BMR. You will also see the food item's SPECIAL FOOD CATEGORY REMINDERS if applicable.

Special Food Category Reminders	
Cx2	**C**ount times **2** – foods are counted twice (page 65)
C/C	**CUP** for **CUP** vegetables – always count towards your **AIM**
FFF	**F**irst **F**ruits **F**ree – your first two fresh fruits in a day do not count
M	**M**eats – lean pref., 4 oz. (113g) **counts (CTS)** as a 1 cup (page 68)
Ø	**NO** count foods and beverages (page 69)

75

"SAMPLE" Daily Menu (1 of 2)

Portion	Breakfast	CUPS
cup or more	WATER [Ø]	0
cup	COFFEE [Ø] or TEA [Ø]	0
1	BANANA [**FFF**]	0
small	BAGEL - 3" diameter (page 122)	0.50
1 pat = tsp.	+ Butter [**Condiment**] (page 79)	0
1	EGG	0.25

Portion	1ˢᵗ Snack	CUPS
cup each	WATER [Ø] plus TEA [Ø]	0
¼ cup = 25	BLUEBERRIES [**FFF**] (page 64 and 149)	0
½	GRANOLA BAR - LFP	0.50

Portion	Lunch	CUPS
cup each	WATER [Ø] plus COFFEE [Ø]	0
½ fruit	½ ORANGE [**FFF**] or ½ APPLE [**FFF**]	0
up to 2 cups	BROCCOLI - steamed [Ø]	0
5 oz.	CHICKEN BREAST - LFP [**M**]	1.25
medium = 3" diam.	POTATO (page 161) – baked [**C/C**]	1

Portion	2ⁿᵈ Snack	CUPS
cup each	WATER [Ø] plus TEA [Ø]	0
¼ cup	STRAWBERRIES [**FFF**]	0
up to 2 cups	CARROTS [Ø]	0

Portion	Dinner	CUPS
cup each	WATER [Ø] plus TEA [Ø]	O
1	VEGETABLE SALAD [Ø]	O
tsp. = 5ml	+ Dressing [**Condiment**] (page 79)	O
2 medium	FLOUR TORTILLAS	1
4 oz.	+ Ground Beef - LFP [**M**]:	1
¼ tsp.	...... Salt [Ø]	O
¼ tbsp.	...... Chili Powder [Ø]	O
¼ cup	...... Onions [Ø]	O
¼ tsp.	...... Minced Garlic [Ø]	O
	+ Salsa Recipe [Ø]:	
7 oz.	...... Diced Tomatoes [Ø]	O
7 oz.	...... Tomatoes + Chiles [Ø]	O
½ tbsp.	...... Lime Juice [Ø]	O
tsp.	...... Minced Garlic [Ø]	O
½ tbsp.	...... Mild Green Chiles [Ø]	O
¼ tsp.	...... Salt [Ø]	O
½ small	...... Diced Onion [Ø]	O
¼ cup	...... Chopped Cilantro [Ø]	O
¼ cup	...... Mango [**FFF**]	O
up to 2 cups	GREEN BEANS [Ø]	O

Next is an example of cup amount entries, based upon the previous **"SAMPLE" Daily Menu**. Tracking by Meal and Tracking by Day have been entered for illustration purposes.

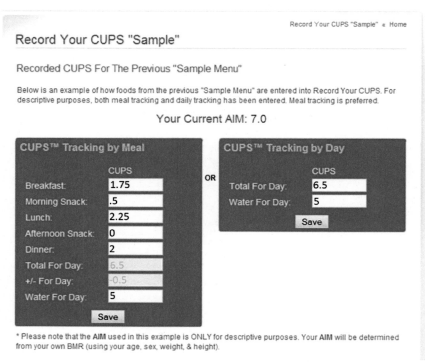

Record Your CUPS "Sample"

Recorded CUPS For The Previous "Sample Menu"

Below is an example of how foods from the previous "Sample Menu" are entered into Record Your CUPS. For descriptive purposes, both meal tracking and daily tracking has been entered. Meal tracking is preferred.

Your Current AIM: 7.0

CUPS™ Tracking by Meal	CUPS			CUPS™ Tracking by Day	CUPS
Breakfast:	1.75		OR	Total For Day:	6.5
Morning Snack:	.5			Water For Day:	5
Lunch:	2.25				Save
Afternoon Snack:	0				
Dinner:	2				
Total For Day:	6.5				
+/- For Day:	-0.5				
Water For Day:	5				
	Save				

* Please note that the AIM used in this example is ONLY for descriptive purposes. Your AIM will be determined from your own BMR (using your age, sex, weight, & height).

*Screenshot "**RECORD YOUR CUPS**" for the SAMPLE Daily Menu,*
from the companion website, www.thecupsdiet.com

At the website select **Using the CUPS diet** tab at the left and you will find **printable PDF files** at the bottom of the drop down menu:

..... **"SAMPLE" Daily Menu**
..... **FOOD APPROXIMATIONS in CUPS**
..... **EXAMPLES of HEALTHY MEALS**
..... **Recipes "From the CUPboard"**

CHAPTER ELEVEN

CONDIMENTS

Next are various condiments and condiment type foods, such as creams and dairy, oils and fats, sauces, spreads and toppings, sugars, and syrups with their Suggested Daily Amount. You may have any item listed, or similar item, in any day and not have to count it toward your **AIM**, that is, if you stay within the Suggested Daily Amount unless noted with [Ø]. If you go over (as listed below), then count that portion of that **Condiment**, as ½ cup toward your **AIM.** For all **Cx2** foods (page 65), count twice if over 2 tablespoons, however with a minimum of ½ cup (noted above).

Suggested Daily Amount of 1 Teaspoon
*For any **condiment**, such as creams and dairy, oils and fats, sauces, spreads and toppings, sugars, and syrups, there is a 1 tsp. suggested daily amount. These will never count toward your* **AIM** *if intake is 1 tsp. or less. If over 1 tsp., count as ½ cup.*

Suggested Daily Amount of 2 Teaspoons
*For any of the following food items there is a 2 tsp. suggested daily amount if it is LOW FAT. These **condiments** will never count toward your* **AIM** *(page 44) if intake is 2 tsp. or less. If over 2 tsp., count as ½ cup.*

Suggested Daily Amount of 2 Tablespoons
*FAT FREE **and** LOW CALORIE **condiments** will never count toward your* **AIM** *if intake is 2 tbsp. or less. If over 2 tbsp., then count as ½ cup.*

Creams [Cx2] and Dairy foods [Cx2] – LFP (Low Fat Preferred):

Butter

Coffee Creamers

Condensed Milk

Evaporated Milk

Grated Cheese

Heavy Cream

Margarine

Sour Cream

Whipping Cream

Half & Half Cream, etc.

Oils [Cx2] and Fats [Cx2] – LFP:

Argan Oil

Canola Oil

Coconut Oil

Corn Oil

Cottonseed Oil

Ghee Oil

Grape Seed Oil

Lard

Olive Oil

Palm or Palm Kernel Oil

Peanut Oil

Pumpkin Seed Oil

Rice Bran Oil

Safflower Oil

Salad Dressing

Sesame Oil

Shortening

Soybean Oil

Sunflower Oil

Vegetable Oil, etc.

Sauces:

BBQ Sauce

Béchamel

Dipping Sauce

Gravy

Horseradish [Ø]

Hoisin

Hot Sauce [Ø]

Ketchup

Marinades

Pesto

Salsa [Ø]

Shrimp Cocktail

Soy Sauce [Ø]

Steak Sauce

Sweet and Sour Sauce

Tartar Sauce

Worcestershire Sauce [Ø]

Spices [Ø] and Herbs [Ø] :

These do not count towards your AIM (page 44).

Spreads and Toppings – LFP (Low Fat Preferred):

Aioli [**Cx2**]
Baba Ghanoush
Butter [**Cx2**]
Capers
Cheese Dips [**Cx2**]
Cheese Spreads [**Cx2**]
Cream **C**heese [**Cx2**]
Chutney
Dairy Spreads
Dips
Fleischbutter
Guacamole
Harissa
Hummus [**Cx2**]
Jam and Jelly [**Cx2**]
Margarine [**Cx2**]
Marmite
Mayonnaise [**Cx2**]
Meat
Mustard [**Ø**]
Nutella
Peanut Butter [**Cx2**]
Pesto
Pickled Ginger
Pico de Gallo [**Ø**]
Relishes
Tapenade
Teriyaki
Vegemite
Vegetable [**Ø**]
Vinegar [**Ø**]
Wasabi [**Ø**], etc.

Sugars [Cx2]:

Brown Sugar
Cane Sugar
Corn Sugar
Honey
Powdered Sugar
Raw Sugar
Semi Sweet Sugar
White Sugar, etc.

Syrups [Cx2] - low calorie preferred:

Agave Nectar
Barley Malt
Brown Rice
Caramel
Chocolate
Corn
Fruit
Fudge
Maple
Molasses
Palm
Sugar Beet, etc.

CHAPTER TWELVE

TIPS for LOSING WEIGHT

COUPLE of CUPS

With **the CUPS diet®** you have flexibility in choosing your foods. Below are key points that will prove invaluable in helping you to enjoy a successful weight loss experience. Vary selections within all of the FOOD GROUPS.

Have up to a **COUPLE** of **CUPS** of .....
..... fresh fruits every day
..... the grains food group every day
Have at least a **COUPLE** of **CUPS** of .....
..... vegetables every day - fresh preferred
..... dairy foods every day - LFP
Have at most a **COUPLE** of **CUPS** of .....
..... protein based foods (meats) every day - LFP

Plus:

Stay within your **AIM** (page 44) and ....

Do not skip any meals or snacks.

Have 3 meals and 2 snacks daily.

Eat breakfast most days of the week.

Eat breakfast within 1 hour of getting up.

Have ½-3 cups for breakfast.

Stay physically active, i.e. walk daily.

Drink 5 glasses of water daily.

Include protein if possible at every meal.

ENJOY your favorite foods.

Do not mistake thirst for hunger.

Add spices for flavor enhancement.

Use **the CUPS diet®** when on a vacation.

Stock your kitchen with healthy foods.

Keep **FFF** (page 67) foods on the table, counter, etc.

Do not eat within 2-3 hours of bedtime.

Get plenty of sleep.

Weigh yourself every week.

Keep track of your daily food intake.

Keep track of your daily exercise.

Visualize your progress.

Limit eating at the TV or computer.

Keep snacks small; 200 calories or less.

Use smaller plates for your meals.

Use **the CUPS diet**® during holidays.

Use larger glasses for your water.

Be sure to set realistic goals.

Do not adopt an all or nothing attitude.

Eat plenty of "**NO** count" vegetables.

ENJOY your favorite food...

.... yes, it bears repeating.

APPENDIX I

FACTORS AFFECTING the BMR

Numerous factors which influence your BMR are listed below. Many interact with each other. Some can be controlled and others are natural processes which we can do little to alter. Four of these factors (age, height, weight, and gender) are used in the BMR calculation itself. BMR can be determined by using a number of different mathematical formulas and procedures. The formula used by **the CUPS diet®** is the Revised Harris-Benedict Equation:

BMR (kcal/day) for men
$$88.362 + (13.397 \times W) + (4.799 \times H) - (5.677 \times A)$$

BMR (kcal/day) for women
$$447.593 + (9.247 \times W) + (3.098 \times H) - (4.33 \times A)$$

W = weight (kg), H = height (cm), A = age (years old.)

*SPECIAL NOTE: When using **the CUPS diet®** it will never be necessary for you to calculate your Basal Metabolic Rate, as this will be done for you automatically with every update in your weight, at the companion website.

1. Age

Our Basal Metabolic Rate will decrease as we age. This is due to loss in muscle tissue, as well as hormonal and neurological changes. Adults have less of a demand for caloric requirements per pound than children as adults need less energy to help support growth needs. BMR will lower by about 0.2-0.3% every year after the age of about thirty. This BMR reduction will inevitably lead to weight gain unless food intake is reduced or physical activity (especially strength training) is increased. In other words, even if you were to remain at the same activity level for your entire life, and you were to eat exactly the same amount of food every day, you would still be prone to weight gain as you age.

the CUPS diet® helps manage the effects of aging as it is related to the gaining of body weight. An appropriate amount of food intake, **AIM** (page 44), that is, your Adjusted Individual Measurement, is recommended based on your current Basal Metabolic Rate.

2. Body Composition

Lean muscle tissue burns calories at a quicker rate than that of adipose (fat) tissue. **the CUPS diet®** helps by reducing fat and increasing the ratio of lean muscle mass, in turn increasing BMR with the resultant continued weight loss.

3. Dietary Restrictions

Excessive weight loss occurs through Starvation, Extreme Dieting (crash), Malnutrition, and even Very Low Calorie Diets (VLCD), and the result is often a large volume of fluid loss. Significant loss of muscle tissue may also be seen with VLCDs. As muscle mass drops, so does the BMR. The body then responds by trying to replace the lost fluids, and weight loss can slow, stop, or even reverse, while metabolism reduces and the body compensates.

The body also will respond to caloric deprivation within about two days, with up to a 45% reduction in the BMR. Extreme (crash) dieting lowers the BMR as much as 15-30%. Diets low in iodine may reduce thyroid function which will also lower the BMR.

"the CUPS diet® *is a Low to Moderate Calorie Diet and does not promote extreme fluid loss or significant muscle tissue loss such as can be seen with Very Low Calorie Diets (VLCDs). The National Heart, Lung, and Blood Institute (NHLBI) have defined VLCDs as diets providing fewer than 800 calories per day".*

4. External Temperature

Extremes of external temperatures tend to produce changes in the BMR. These changes can be about 5-20% higher than those found in moderate temperatures. In tropical settings the BMR can actually decrease by as much as 20%. Extreme external temperatures can also increase the internal body temperature. An increase of one degree in body temperature (in Centigrade) can raise the BMR as much as 13%. In arctic conditions, the Basal Metabolic Rate can increase by as much as 20%.

5. Gender

Females will usually have a lower BMR (by 5-10%) than males, due to the fact that females usually have a lower percentage of lean body mass than males. This is not always the case, however, as women can have a higher percentage (especially female athletes), and thus a higher Basal Metabolic Rate.

6. Height

Total body surface area exposure is partially determined by height and thus, height is a factor in calculating an individual's Basal Metabolic Rate. This is due to the fact that a tall individual has a larger exposure of skin surface and thus will experience a higher rate of heat loss from the body. This must be compensated for by a higher Basal Metabolic Rate.

7. Hormones

The thyroid hormones, thyroxin (T4) in particular, as well as triiodothyronine (T3) can affect the BMR. In hypothyroidism (underactive thyroid) weight gain can occur due to a reduction in the BMR. There is also an increased risk in women for hypothyroidism, near or after menopause. Stress related hormones, such as epinephrine (adrenaline), norepinephrine and cortisol can also influence an individual's BMR. Testosterone levels can affect the BMR and, because women have only about 5-10% of the levels as men, they are more likely to experience weight gain due to having less muscle mass.

8. Menstruation

About two weeks before menstruation begins, it is not unusual to see an increase in food intake due to an increased appetite. During menstruation, BMR increases by about 10%, but this increase does not offset the increased food consumption. Food intake must be controlled or weight gain will occur.

9. Overall Health Status

Fevers and illnesses can increase body temperature. As noted previously in "External Temperature" an increase of one degree of body temperature can raise the Basal Metabolic Rate by up to 13%.

10. Physical Activity

Caloric restrictions alone reduce the Basal Metabolic Rate. However when physical activity is added, this lower BMR will begin to increase again. Metabolism increases for up to twenty four hours after physical activity, and is dependent upon the level of that activity. Therefore it is not uncommon to experience a period of slower weight loss as fat is lost and replaced by muscle tissue, which weighs more. As muscle becomes more prominent with lean body mass, an increase in BMR occurs because lean body mass burns calories at a higher rate than non-lean tissues.

To assist with your weight loss, try 30 minutes of moderate physical activity (beyond your normal routine) most days of the week. Appropriate activities may include; walking, jogging, running, weight lifting, swimming, or biking. These recommendations are from the 1996 Surgeon General's report on Physical Activity and Health and are stressed in the Dietary Guidelines for Americans 2005, from the Department of Health & Human Services and the Department of Agriculture. It is also recommended that, whatever type of exercise you choose, a diary be kept of your activities.

11. Weight

As body weight increases, cardiovascular and respiratory systems must work harder to support more mass. This results in the need for additional caloric intake and an increase in BMR. The converse is also true in that as weight is lost, BMR will decrease. With **the CUPS diet**® the food intake recommended will adjust based on this new BMR so as to assist with further weight loss.

APPENDIX II

EXAMPLES of HEALTHY MEALS

Following are a number of menu examples with a nutritional breakdown for **the CUPS diet**® compiled with the assistance of PerLa Nancy González Salazar, Registered Dietician, Monterrey, Nuevo León, Mexico. These 26 examples amply demonstrate how simple meal planning can be and how to count certain foods. At the website you can **print PDF files** of these meals. The symbols below will follow any special food/beverage as a reminder of special instructions to be used in determining food intake.

Breakfast Examples
2 cup (5)
3 cup (2)
Lunch Examples
2 cup (4)
2½ cup (1)
3 cup (1)
Dinner Examples
2 cup (7)
Snacks Examples
½ cup (6)

Special Food Category Reminders	
Cx2	**C**ount times **2** – foods are counted twice (page 65)
C/C	**CUP** for **CUP** vegetables – always count towards your **AIM**
FFF	**F**irst **F**ruits **F**ree – your first two fresh fruits in a day do not count
LFP	**L**ow **F**at **P**referred
M	**M**eats – lean pref., 4 oz. (113g) **counts (CTS)** as a 1 cup (page 68)
∅	**NO** count foods and beverages (page 69)

2 cup BREAKFAST EXAMPLES .....

Portion	Breakfast – menu #1	CUPS
cup	WATER [∅]	0
cup	COFFEE [∅] or TEA [∅] is optional	0
¼ cup = 1 oz.	BLUEBERRIES [FFF] (page 64 & 149)	0
small = 1-3" diameter	BAGEL (page 122)	0.50
1 oz.	+ Cream Cheese [Cx2] is ¼ cup x2	0.50
	FRUIT SMOOTHIE:	
cup	..... Skim Milk	1
¼ cup = 5 small	..... Strawberries [FFF]	0

CUPS, Weight, and Diameter Equivalents (page 61)

Nutritional Facts / Datos de Nutrición	
Calories / Calorias:	378
Total Fat / Todo de Grasa:	10.8g
Sat Fat / Grasa Sat:	6.4g
Trans Fat / Grasa Trans:	0
Cholesterol / Colesterol:	35mg
Sodium / Sodo:	461mg
Total Carb / Todo de Carbohidratos:	53g
Dietary Fiber / Fibra Dietética:	2.7g
Sugars / Azúcar:	20.3g
Protein / Proteínas:	16.6g
Calcium / Calcio:	32.4mg
Potassium / Potasio:	509mg

2 cup BREAKFAST EXAMPLES (cont.)

Portion	Breakfast – menu #2	CUPS
cup	WATER [Ø]	O
cup	COFFEE [Ø] is optional	O
cup	TEA [Ø] is optional	O
2-4 oz.	MUSHROOMS [Ø]	O
2	EGG WHITES - cooked	0.25
slice	TOAST - whole wheat preferred	0.50
1¼ cup = 10 fl. oz.	ORANGE JUICE	1.25

CUPS, Weight, and Diameter Equivalents (page 61)

Nutritional Facts / Datos de Nutrición	
Calories / Calorias:	245
Total Fat / Todo de Grasa:	1.7g
Sat Fat / Grasa Sat:	0.1g
Trans Fat / Grasa Trans:	O
Cholesterol / Colesterol:	O
Sodium / Sodo:	185mg
Total Carb / Todo de Carbohidratos:	45.5g
Dietary Fiber / Fibra Dietética:	4.1g
Sugars / Azúcar:	28g
Protein / Proteínas:	13.4g
Calcium / Calcio:	48.3mg
Potassium / Potasio:	809.5mg

2 cup BREAKFAST EXAMPLES (cont.)

Portion	Breakfast – menu #3	CUPS
cup	WATER [Ø]	O
cup	COFFEE [Ø] is optional	O
cup	TEA [Ø] is optional	O
¼ cup = 1 oz.	BLUEBERRIES [FFF] (page 64 & 149)	O
¼ cup = 5 small	STRAWBERRIES [FFF]	O
cup	MILK - LFP	1
1 = 2-4" diameter	PANCAKES – without syrup	1

CUPS, Weight, and Diameter Equivalents (page 61)

Nutritional Facts / Datos de Nutrición	
Calories / Calorias:	317
Total Fat / Todo de Grasa:	3g
Sat Fat / Grasa Sat:	0.8g
Trans Fat / Grasa Trans:	O
Cholesterol / Colesterol:	5mg
Sodium / Sodo:	611mg
Total Carb / Todo de Carbohidratos:	60g
Dietary Fiber / Fibra Dietética:	4.1g
Sugars / Azúcar:	25.6g
Protein / Proteínas:	13.7g
Calcium / Calcio:	427.9mg
Potassium / Potasio:	718mg

2 cup BREAKFAST EXAMPLES (cont.)

Portion	Breakfast — menu #4	CUPS
cup	WATER [Ø]	O
cup	COFFEE [Ø] is optional	O
cup	TEA [Ø] is optional	O
	BREAKFAST MILKSHAKE:	
any size	..... Banana [FFF]	O
cup	..... Milk - LFP	1
2	WAFFLES	1
tsp.	+ low calorie syrup [Ø]	O

CUPS, Weight, and Diameter Equivalents (page 61)

Nutritional Facts / Datos de Nutrición	
Calories / *Calorias:*	**240**
Total Fat / *Todo de Grasa:*	2.6g
Sat Fat / *Grasa Sat:*	0.8g
Trans Fat / *Grasa Trans:*	O
Cholesterol / *Colesterol:*	14mg
Sodium / *Sodo:*	607mg
Total Carb / *Todo de Carbohidratos:*	40g
Dietary Fiber / *Fibra Dietética:*	3g
Sugars / *Azúcar:*	14g
Protein / *Proteínas:*	12.7g
Calcium / *Calcio:*	412mg
Potassium / *Potasio:*	712mg

2 cup BREAKFAST EXAMPLES (cont.)

Portion	Breakfast – menu #5	CUPS
cup	WATER [∅]	0
cup	COFFEE [∅] is optional	0
cup	TEA [∅] is optional	0
2 cups	MIXED FRUITS [FFF]	0
slice	TOAST - whole wheat preferred	0.50
2 tsp.	+ Peanut Butter – low fat	0.50
½ cup = 4 oz.	YOGURT – fat free preferred	0.50
½ cup = 5 cashews	CASHEWS [Cx2] is ¼ cup x2	0.50

CUPS, Weight, and Diameter Equivalents (page 61)

Nutritional Facts / Datos de Nutrición	
Calories / Calorias:	250
Total Fat / Todo de Grasa:	8.5g
Sat Fat / Grasa Sat:	1.9g
Trans Fat / Grasa Trans:	0
Cholesterol / Colesterol:	5mg
Sodium / Sodo:	200mg
Total Carb / Todo de Carbohidratos:	35g
Dietary Fiber / Fibra Dietética:	3g
Sugars / Azúcar:	26.7g
Protein / Proteínas:	16.6g
Calcium / Calcio:	495mg
Potassium / Potasio:	740mg

3 cup BREAKFAST EXAMPLES .....

Portion	Breakfast — menu #6	CUPS
cup	WATER [Ø]	O
cup	COFFEE [Ø] is optional	O
cup	TEA [Ø] is optional	O
¾ cup = 6 fl. oz.	MILK - LFP	0.75
any size	APPLE [FFF]	O
2 slices	TOAST SANDWICH:	1
slice each	..... Lettuce [Ø] & Tomato [Ø]	O
slice or 1 oz.	..... Meat — LFP [M]	0.25
slice or 1 oz.	..... Cheese [Cx2] is ¼ cup x2	0.50
½ cup = 4 oz.	YOGURT — LFP	0.50

CUPS, Weight, and Diameter Equivalents (page 61)

Nutritional Facts / *Datos de Nutrición*	
Calories / *Calorias:*	**396**
Total Fat / *Todo de Grasa:*	9.8g
Sat Fat / *Grasa Sat:*	4.4g
Trans Fat / *Grasa Trans:*	O
Cholesterol / *Colesterol:*	41mg
Sodium / *Sodo:*	796mg
Total Carb / *Todo de Carbohidratos:*	53.7g
Dietary Fiber / *Fibra Dietética:*	9.6g
Sugars / *Azúcar:*	20.2g
Protein / *Proteínas:*	17.2g
Calcium / *Calcio:*	541.9mg
Potassium / *Potasio:*	462.1mg

3 cup BREAKFAST EXAMPLES (cont.)

Portion	Breakfast — menu #7	CUPS
cup	WATER [Ø]	O
cup	COFFEE [Ø] is optional	O
cup	TEA [Ø] is optional	O
any size	BANANA [FFF]	O
cup (cooked)	OATMEAL - or ½ cup dry	1
packet	+ Artificial Sweetener [Ø]	O
tbsp. = 1 oz.	NUTS [Cx2] is ¼ cup x2	0.50
2 slices	TOAST - whole wheat preferred	1
slice or 1 oz.	+ Cheese [Cx2] is ¼ cup x2	0.50

CUPS, Weight, and Diameter Equivalents (page 61)

Nutritional Facts / Datos de Nutrición	
Calories / Calorias:	350
Total Fat / Todo de Grasa:	12.5g
Sat Fat / Grasa Sat:	1.4g
Trans Fat / Grasa Trans:	O
Cholesterol / Colesterol:	O
Sodium / Sodo:	3mg
Total Carb / Todo de Carbohidratos:	77g
Dietary Fiber / Fibra Dietética:	8.5g
Sugars / Azúcar:	17.6g
Protein / Proteínas:	9.9g
Calcium / Calcio:	40.2mg
Potassium / Potasio:	684mg

2 cup LUNCH EXAMPLES .....

Portion	Lunch — menu #8	CUPS
cup	WATER [Ø]	O
cup	COFFEE [Ø] is optional	O
cup	TEA [Ø] is optional	O
cup	BROCCOLI – steamed [Ø]	O
4 oz.	CHICKEN BREAST - skinless [M]	1
medium	POTATO - baked [C/C]	1

CUPS, Weight, and Diameter Equivalents (page 61)

Nutritional Facts / Datos de Nutrición	
Calories / Calorias:	346
Total Fat / Todo de Grasa:	2.3g
Sat Fat / Grasa Sat:	0.5g
Trans Fat / Grasa Trans:	< 0.1g
Cholesterol / Colesterol:	66mg
Sodium / Sodo:	147mg
Total Carb / Todo de Carbohidratos:	48g
Dietary Fiber / Fibra Dietética:	9.1g
Sugars / Azúcar:	6.4g
Protein / Proteínas:	34.7g
Calcium / Calcio:	101.8mg
Potassium / Potasio:	1,516.9mg

2 cup LUNCH EXAMPLES (cont.)

Portion	Lunch – menu #9	CUPS
cup	WATER [Ø]	O
cup	COFFEE [Ø] is optional	O
cup	TEA [Ø] is optional	O
cup (cooked)	PASTA – or 2 oz. dry	1
cup	VEGETABLES – fresh [Ø]	O
4 oz. = 5 large	SHRIMP [M]	1

CUPS, Weight, and Diameter Equivalents (page 61)

Nutritional Facts / *Datos de Nutrición*	
Calories / *Calorias:*	**420**
Total Fat / *Todo de Grasa:*	2.7g
Sat Fat / *Grasa Sat:*	0.5g
Trans Fat / *Grasa Trans:*	O
Cholesterol / *Colesterol:*	38mg
Sodium / *Sodo:*	282mg
Total Carb / *Todo de Carbohidratos:*	76.7g
Dietary Fiber / *Fibra Dietética:*	8.5g
Sugars / *Azúcar:*	5.1g
Protein / *Proteínas:*	20.8g
Calcium / *Calcio:*	70.9mg
Potassium / *Potasio:*	609.9mg

2 cup LUNCH EXAMPLES (cont.)

Portion	Lunch – menu #10	CUPS
cup	WATER [⊘]	O
cup	COFFEE [⊘] is optional	O
cup	TEA [⊘] is optional	O
	SALAD:	
1	..... Under 6 Veggie Delight	O
6"	SUBWAY SANDWICH – all types	2

CUPS, Weight, and Diameter Equivalents (page 61)

Nutritional Facts / *Datos de Nutrición*	
Calories / *Calorias:*	**350**
Total Fat / *Todo de Grasa:*	7g
Sat Fat / *Grasa Sat:*	1g
Trans Fat / *Grasa Trans:*	O
Cholesterol / *Colesterol:*	20mg
Sodium / *Sodo:*	1,000mg
Total Carb / *Todo de Carbohidratos:*	52g
Dietary Fiber / *Fibra Dietética:*	7g
Sugars / *Azúcar:*	7g
Protein / *Proteínas:*	21g
Calcium / *Calcio:*	80mg
Potassium / *Potasio:*	O

2 cup LUNCH EXAMPLES (cont.)

Portion	Lunch – menu #11	CUPS
cup	WATER [Ø]	O
cup	COFFEE [Ø] is optional	O
cup	TEA [Ø] is optional	O
4 oz.	FISH FILLET – grilled [M]	1
2 cups	GREEN SALAD [Ø]	O
4 oz. (cooked)	RICE - or 2 oz. dry	1

CUPS, Weight, and Diameter Equivalents (page 61)

Nutritional Facts / Datos de Nutrición	
Calories / Calorias:	352
Total Fat / Todo de Grasa:	4.3g
Sat Fat / Grasa Sat:	0.6g
Trans Fat / Grasa Trans:	O
Cholesterol / Colesterol:	55mg
Sodium / Sodo:	101mg
Total Carb / Todo de Carbohidratos:	35g
Dietary Fiber / Fibra Dietética:	1.5g
Sugars / Azúcar:	0.1g
Protein / Proteínas:	40.1g
Calcium / Calcio:	111mg
Potassium / Potasio:	119.7mg

2½ cup LUNCH EXAMPLE .....

Portion	Lunch – menu #12	CUPS
cup	WATER [∅]	O
cup	COFFEE [∅] is optional	O
cup	TEA [∅] is optional	O
2 cups	VEGETABLE SALAD - fresh [∅]	O
tsp.	+ Salad Dressing [tsp = ∅]	O
½ cup = 4 oz.	PUDDING – LFP	0.50
2 slices	PIZZA – thin	2

CUPS, Weight, and Diameter Equivalents (page 61)

Nutritional Facts / *Datos de Nutrición*	
Calories / *Calorias:*	**430**
Total Fat / *Todo de Grasa:*	20.6g
Sat Fat / *Grasa Sat:*	5.5g
Trans Fat / *Grasa Trans:*	< 0.1g
Cholesterol / *Colesterol:*	9.3mg
Sodium / *Sodo:*	1,586mg
Total Carb / *Todo de Carbohidratos:*	57.9g
Dietary Fiber / *Fibra Dietética:*	5g
Sugars / *Azúcar:*	3.7g
Protein / *Proteínas:*	12.4g
Calcium / *Calcio:*	80.3mg
Potassium / *Potasio:*	126.1mg

3 cup LUNCH EXAMPLE .....

Portion	Lunch – menu #13	CUPS
cup	WATER [Ø]	O
cup	COFFEE [Ø] is optional	O
cup	TEA [Ø] is optional	O
	VEGETABLE SOUP:	
cup	..... Broth [Ø]	O
cup	..... **NO** count Fresh Vegetables [Ø]	O
1	GRANOLA BAR – LFP	1
1	STUFFED BURRITO - grilled	2

CUPS, Weight, and Diameter Equivalents (page 61)

Nutritional Facts / *Datos de Nutrición*	
Calories / *Calorias:*	**450**
Total Fat / *Todo de Grasa:*	9.5g
Sat Fat / *Grasa Sat:*	2.5g
Trans Fat / *Grasa Trans:*	O
Cholesterol / *Colesterol:*	75mg
Sodium / *Sodo:*	1,140mg
Total Carb / *Todo de Carbohidratos:*	69g
Dietary Fiber / *Fibra Dietética:*	8g
Sugars / *Azúcar:*	11g
Protein / *Proteínas:*	19g
Calcium / *Calcio:*	80mg
Potassium / *Potasio:*	200mg

2 cup DINNER EXAMPLES .....

Portion	Dinner – menu #14	CUPS
cup	WATER [Ø]	O
cup	COFFEE [Ø] is optional	O
cup	TEA [Ø] is optional	O
1¼ cup = 10 oz.	SOUP – LFP	1.25
½	AVOCADO [FFF]	O
1-2 tsp.	+ Fresh Squeezed Lime Juice [FFF]	O
2	SALTINE CRACKERS	0.25
½ cup	TUNA SALAD	0.50

CUPS, Weight, and Diameter Equivalents (page 61)

Nutritional Facts / Datos de Nutrición	
Calories / Calorias:	460
Total Fat / Todo de Grasa:	12.9g
Sat Fat / Grasa Sat:	2g
Trans Fat / Grasa Trans:	O
Cholesterol / Colesterol:	35mg
Sodium / Sodo:	1,147mg
Total Carb / Todo de Carbohidratos:	34.75g
Dietary Fiber / Fibra Dietética:	11.45g
Sugars / Azúcar:	1.7g
Protein / Proteínas:	25g
Calcium / Calcio:	35mg
Potassium / Potasio:	487.4mg

2 cup DINNER EXAMPLES (cont.)

Portion	Dinner – menu #15	CUPS
cup	WATER [Ø]	0
cup	COFFEE [Ø] is optional	0
cup	TEA [Ø] is optional	0
½	GRANOLA BAR – LFP	1
4 oz.	CHICKEN CAESAR - grilled	1

CUPS, Weight, and Diameter Equivalents (page 61)

Nutritional Facts / Datos de Nutrición	
Calories / Calorias:	**320**
Total Fat / Todo de Grasa:	9g
Sat Fat / Grasa Sat:	3.3g
Trans Fat / Grasa Trans:	0
Cholesterol / Colesterol:	75mg
Sodium / Sodo:	970mg
Total Carb / Todo de Carbohidratos:	26.5g
Dietary Fiber / Fibra Dietética:	4g
Sugars / Azúcar:	10.5g
Protein / Proteínas:	32g
Calcium / Calcio:	200mg
Potassium / Potasio:	316-394mg

2 cup DINNER EXAMPLES (cont.)

Portion	Snack — menu #16	CUPS
cup	WATER [Ø]	O
cup	COFFEE [Ø] is optional	O
cup	TEA [Ø] is optional	O
2 cups	LETTUCE SALAD [Ø]	O
3 slices	+ Onion [Ø] & Tomato [Ø]	O
2 tsp.	+ Cranberry Balsamic Vinegar [Ø]	O
2 tsp.	+ Olive Oil [**Condiment**] (page 79)	0.50
2	+ English Walnuts [**Cx2**] is ¼ cup **x2**	0.50
2 oz.	+ Goat Cheese [**Cx2**] is ½ cup **x2**	1

CUPS, Weight, and Diameter Equivalents (page 61)

Nutritional Facts / *Datos de Nutrición*	
Calories / *Calorias:*	**477**
Total Fat / *Todo de Grasa:*	39.4g
Sat Fat / *Grasa Sat:*	10.9g
Trans Fat / *Grasa Trans:*	O
Cholesterol / *Colesterol:*	40mg
Sodium / *Sodo:*	47mg
Total Carb / *Todo de Carbohidratos:*	16.6g
Dietary Fiber / *Fibra Dietética:*	4.1g
Sugars / *Azúcar:*	9.4g
Protein / *Proteínas:*	16.6g
Calcium / *Calcio:*	177.7mg
Potassium / *Potasio:*	459.8mg

2 cup DINNER EXAMPLES (cont.)

Portion	Dinner – menu #17	CUPS
cup	WATER [∅]	0
cup	COFFEE [∅] is optional	0
cup	TEA [∅] is optional	0
10 pieces	SUSHI ROLL – cold	2

CUPS, Weight, and Diameter Equivalents (page 61)

Nutritional Facts / *Datos de Nutrición*	
Calories / *Calorias:*	**365**
Total Fat / *Todo de Grasa:*	5g
Sat Fat / *Grasa Sat:*	1g
Trans Fat / *Grasa Trans:*	0
Cholesterol / *Colesterol:*	0
Sodium / *Sodo:*	1,182mg
Total Carb / *Todo de Carbohidratos:*	70g
Dietary Fiber / *Fibra Dietética:*	3g
Sugars / *Azúcar:*	13g
Protein / *Proteínas:*	8g
Calcium / *Calcio:*	60mg
Potassium / *Potasio:*	0-340mg

2 cup DINNER EXAMPLES (cont.)

Portion	Dinner — menu #18	CUPS
cup	WATER [∅]	0
cup	COFFEE [∅] is optional	0
cup	TEA [∅] is optional	0
cup	VEGETABLES - fresh [∅]	0
large = 3" diameter	POTATO (page 161) - baked [C/C]	1
1 oz.	+ Cream Cheese [Cx2] is ¼ cup x2	0.50
¼ cup = 5 small	STRAWBERRIES [FFF] (page 64 & 149)	0
½ cup = 4 oz.	YOGURT – LFP	0.50

CUPS, Weight, and Diameter Equivalents (page 61)

Nutritional Facts / Datos de Nutrición	
Calories / Calorias:	507
Total Fat / Todo de Grasa:	11g
Sat Fat / Grasa Sat:	6.3g
Trans Fat / Grasa Trans:	0
Cholesterol / Colesterol:	32mg
Sodium / Sodo:	908mg
Total Carb / Todo de Carbohidratos:	86.9g
Dietary Fiber / Fibra Dietética:	8.4g
Sugars / Azúcar:	13.7g
Protein / Proteínas:	19.8g
Calcium / Calcio:	315.9mg
Potassium / Potasio:	2,446.3mg

2 cup DINNER EXAMPLES (cont.)

Portion	Dinner – menu #19	CUPS
cup	WATER [∅]	0
cup	COFFEE [∅] is optional	0
cup	TEA [∅] is optional	0
	SHRIMP QUESADILLAS:	
½ cup	..... Sliced Peppers [∅]	0
10 medium = 2 oz.	..... Shrimp [M]	0.50
slice or 1 oz.	..... Cheese [Cx2] is ¼ cup x2	0.50
2 medium	..... Corn Tortillas	1

CUPS, Weight, and Diameter Equivalents (page 61)

Nutritional Facts / Datos de Nutrición	
Calories / Calorias:	**193**
Total Fat / Todo de Grasa:	5.8g
Sat Fat / Grasa Sat:	3g
Trans Fat / Grasa Trans:	0
Cholesterol / Colesterol:	61mg
Sodium / Sodo:	235mg
Total Carb / Todo de Carbohidratos:	20.9g
Dietary Fiber / Fibra Dietética:	3.8g
Sugars / Azúcar:	3.4g
Protein / Proteínas:	13.9g
Calcium / Calcio:	28.6mg
Potassium / Potasio:	164.3mg

2 cup DINNER EXAMPLES (cont.)

Portion	Dinner — menu #20	CUPS
cup	WATER [Ø]	O
cup	TEA [Ø] is optional	O
2 cups	VEGETABLE SALAD [Ø]	O
tsp.	+ Salad Dressing [tsp = Ø]	O
4 oz.	GROUND BEEF – LFP [M]	1
½ cup = 4 oz.	+ Mushrooms [Ø]	O
cup (cooked)	PASTA – or 2 oz. dry	1
½ cup = 4 oz.	+ Marinara Sauce [Ø]	O

CUPS, Weight, and Diameter Equivalents (page 61)

Nutritional Facts / Datos de Nutrición	
Calories / Calorias:	550
Total Fat / Todo de Grasa:	16g
Sat Fat / Grasa Sat:	3.7g
Trans Fat / Grasa Trans:	0.2g
Cholesterol / Colesterol:	365mg
Sodium / Sodo:	272mg
Total Carb / Todo de Carbohidratos:	61.5g
Dietary Fiber / Fibra Dietética:	4g
Sugars / Azúcar:	2.7g
Protein / Proteínas:	39.4g
Calcium / Calcio:	59.6mg
Potassium / Potasio:	576mg

½ cup SNACK EXAMPLES .....

Portion	Snack – menu #21	CUPS
cup	WATER [⊘]	O
cup	COFFEE [⊘] is optional	O
cup	TEA [⊘] is optional	O
½ mini bag	POPCORN - 94% fat free	O.5O

CUPS, Weight, and Diameter Equivalents (page 61)

Nutritional Facts / *Datos de Nutrición*	
Calories / *Calorias:*	**1OO**
Total Fat / *Todo de Grasa:*	1.5g
Sat Fat / *Grasa Sat:*	O
Trans Fat / *Grasa Trans:*	O
Cholesterol / *Colesterol:*	O
Sodium / *Sodo:*	170mg
Total Carb / *Todo de Carbohidratos:*	21g
Dietary Fiber / *Fibra Dietética:*	3g
Sugars / *Azúcar:*	O
Protein / *Proteínas:*	3g
Calcium / *Calcio:*	O
Potassium / *Potasio:*	79.5mg

½ cup SNACK EXAMPLES (cont.)

Portion	Snack – menu #22	CUPS
cup	WATER [⦸]	0
cup	COFFEE [⦸] is optional	0
cup	TEA [⦸] is optional	0
½ cup = 4 oz.	PUDDING – fat free	0.50

CUPS, Weight, and Diameter Equivalents (page 61)

Nutritional Facts / Datos de Nutrición	
Calories / Calorias:	102
Total Fat / Todo de Grasa:	0.5g
Sat Fat / Grasa Sat:	0.3g
Trans Fat / Grasa Trans:	0
Cholesterol / Colesterol:	2g
Sodium / Sodo:	192mg
Total Carb / Todo de Carbohidratos:	22.7g
Dietary Fiber / Fibra Dietética:	0.9g
Sugars / Azúcar:	17.3g
Protein / Proteínas:	2.8g
Calcium / Calcio:	200mg
Potassium / Potasio:	0

½ cup SNACK EXAMPLES (cont.)

Portion	Snack – menu #23	CUPS
cup	WATER [Ø]	O
cup	COFFEE [Ø] is optional	O
cup	TEA [Ø] is optional	O
100 cal. Snack Pack	HONEY MAID GRAHAMS	0.50

CUPS, Weight, and Diameter Equivalents (page 61)

Nutritional Facts / *Datos de Nutrición*	
Calories / *Calorias:*	**100**
Total Fat / *Todo de Grasa:*	2g
Sat Fat / *Grasa Sat:*	O
Trans Fat / *Grasa Trans:*	O
Cholesterol / *Colesterol:*	O
Sodium / *Sodo:*	170mg
Total Carb / *Todo de Carbohidratos:*	19g
Dietary Fiber / *Fibra Dietética:*	1g
Sugars / *Azúcar:*	7g
Protein / *Proteínas:*	1g
Calcium / *Calcio:*	20mg
Potassium / *Potasio:*	O

½ cup SNACK EXAMPLES (cont.)

Portion	Snack – menu #24	CUPS
cup	WATER [Ø]	0
cup	COFFEE [Ø] is optional	0
cup	TEA [Ø] is optional	0
½	GRANOLA BAR – LFP	0.50

CUPS, Weight, and Diameter Equivalents (page 61)

Nutritional Facts / Datos de Nutrición	
Calories / *Calorias:*	**45**
Total Fat / *Todo de Grasa:*	1.5g
Sat Fat / *Grasa Sat:*	0.3g
Trans Fat / *Grasa Trans:*	0
Cholesterol / *Colesterol:*	0
Sodium / *Sodo:*	40mg
Total Carb / *Todo de Carbohidratos:*	0.5g
Dietary Fiber / *Fibra Dietética:*	3.5g
Sugars / *Azúcar:*	21g
Protein / *Proteínas:*	5g
Calcium / *Calcio:*	0
Potassium / *Potasio:*	0

½ cup SNACK EXAMPLES (cont.)

Portion	Snack – menu #25	CUPS
cup	WATER [∅]	O
cup	COFFEE [∅] is optional	O
cup	TEA [∅] is optional	O
½ cup	SOUP – fat free	0.50
¼ cup = 5 small	STRAWBERRIES [FFF] (page 64 & 149)	O
½ cup = 4 oz.	YOGURT - LFP	0.50

CUPS, Weight, and Diameter Equivalents (page 61)

Nutritional Facts / Datos de Nutrición	
Calories / Calorias:	87
Total Fat / Todo de Grasa:	0.4g
Sat Fat / Grasa Sat:	0.2g
Trans Fat / Grasa Trans:	O
Cholesterol / Colesterol:	2mg
Sodium / Sodo:	88mg
Total Carb / Todo de Carbohidratos:	14.2g
Dietary Fiber / Fibra Dietética:	1.4g
Sugars / Azúcar:	9.2g
Protein / Proteínas:	7g
Calcium / Calcio:	237.2mg
Potassium / Potasio:	399.4mg

½ cup SNACK EXAMPLES (cont.)

Portion	Snack – menu #26	CUPS
cup	WATER [◉]	0
cup	COFFEE [◉] is optional	0
cup	TEA [◉] is optional	0
½ cup = 4 oz.	SOUP – fat free	0.50

CUPS, Weight, and Diameter Equivalents (page 61)

Nutritional Facts / Datos de Nutrición	
Calories / Calorias:	**40**
Total Fat / Todo de Grasa:	0
Sat Fat / Grasa Sat:	0
Trans Fat / Grasa Trans:	0
Cholesterol / Colesterol:	0
Sodium / Sodo:	230mg
Total Carb / Todo de Carbohidratos:	7.5g
Dietary Fiber / Fibra Dietética:	1.5g
Sugars / Azúcar:	0
Protein / Proteínas:	2g
Calcium / Calcio:	0
Potassium / Potasio:	0

APPENDIX III

FOOD APPROXIMATIONS in CUPS

Next are foods and beverages with "CUP" amount for the portions indicated. Note that not every type of food is listed. If something you want to eat is not on this list, you can still enjoy it using **the CUPS diet**®. To assist weight loss it is suggested that no more than a **COUPLE** of **CUPS** of any one food be eaten at any meal.

At the website you can **print PDF files** of these tables.

Low fat and/or low calorie foods are encouraged, but never required. You need to enjoy what you eat, and with **the CUPS diet**® you will.

In these tables there are numerous foods that contain specific **Cx2** foods (page 65). As an aid in remembering the foods in this category, recall that many of the **Cx2** foods also begin with the letter "**C**", such as the "**C**heese" in "**C**heeseburger". The "CUP" amounts of these foods have already been taken into account and you do not need to count them twice, unless it specifically shows the reminder "**x2**" after the food item.

Additional Reminders

Special Food Category Reminders	
Cx2	**C**ount times **2** – foods are counted twice (page 65)
C/C	**CUP** for **CUP** vegetables – always count towards your **AIM**
FFF	**F**irst **F**ruits **F**ree – your first two fresh fruits in a day do not count
M	**M**eats – lean preferred, 4 oz. (113g) **counts (CTS)** as 1 cup (page 68)
Ø	**NO** count foods and beverages (page 69)

117

BEVERAGES

Human nature dictates that when using a large container for a beverage, we tend to drink more than appropriate. To help limit intake use a glass that will hold ½-¾ of a cup when drinking anything other than water.

BEVERAGES - Alcohol

Portion	Alcohol	CUPS
1½ cups	BEER:	1.50
1½ cups	**.... Light**	1
shot = 1.5 fl. oz.	LIQUOR	0.50
cup	MIXED DRINKS	1
cup	+ using diet mix	0
¾ cup	WINE	0.75
CUPS, Weight, and Diameter Equivalents (page 61)		

*There is an exception regarding beer. Twelve fluid ounces of **Light** beer will count as 1 cup. Alcohol should always be used in moderation.*
www.cdc.gov/alcohol/faqs.htm

BEVERAGES - Coffee and Tea

Portion	Coffee [∅] and Tea [∅]	CUPS
cup	CAFÉ AMERICANO [∅]	0
cup	COFFEE [∅] and TEA [∅]	0
tsp.	+ Creamer – LFP [Condiment] (page 79)	0
packet	+ Artificial Sweetener [∅]	0
packet or tsp.	+ Sugar [Condiment]	0
>2 tsp. of one	+ Sugar or Creamer – LFP	0.50
>2 tsp. of both	+ Sugar and Creamer – LFP	1
cup	CAFÉ LATTE [Cx2] is 1 cup x2	2
cup	CAPPUCCINO [Cx2] is 1 cup x2	2
cup	ESPRESSO [∅]	0
cup	ICED COFFEE [∅]	0
cup	MACCHIOTA [Cx2] is 1 cup x2	2
cup	MOCHA [Cx2] is 1 cup x2	2
cup	.... Caramel	2
cup	.... Frapucino	2
cup	.... Frappé (includes Iced)	2
CUPS, Weight, and Diameter Equivalents (page 61)		

Coffee or Tea (with or without caffeine) does not count toward your AIM (page 44). Try to limit your intake to 2 caffeinated a day and de-caffeinated thereafter.

BEVERAGES - Juice and Milk

Portion	JUICE	CUPS
cup	FRUIT JUICE - all types	1
cup	TOMATO - low salt preferred [Ø]	O*
cup	VEGETABLE - low salt preferred [Ø]	O*
cup	V8 JUICE - low salt preferred [Ø]	O*
CUPS, Weight, and Diameter Equivalents (page 61)		

Up to one cup a day of Vegetable, V8, or Tomato Juice (low salt preferred) which will not count toward your AIM (page 44).

Portion	Milk - LFP	CUPS
cup	ALMOND MILK	1
cup	COCONUT MILK [Cx2] is 1 cup x2	2
cup	MALTED MILK [Cx2] is 1 cup x2	2
cup	MILK – including:	1
¼ cup	.... Condensed Milk [Cx2] is ¼ cup x2	0.50
cup	.... Cow Milk or Goat Milk or Sheep Milk, etc.	1
¼ cup	.... Evaporated Milk [Cx2] is ¼ cup x2	0.50
cup	MILKSHAKE [Cx2] is 1 cup x2	2
cup	RICE MILK	1
cup	SOY MILK	1
CUPS, Weight, and Diameter Equivalents (page 61)		

BEVERAGES – Protein and Soda and Water

Protein Mix (added to water)	CUPS
Divide calories by 200 (then round it to the nearest ¼ increment)	
..... example #1. 160/200 = 0.80, round to →	0.75
..... example #2. 120/200 = 0.60, round to →	0.50

Portion	Soda	CUPS
1½ cups	DIET SODA [Ø]	0
1½ cups	LOW CALORIE	0.50
1½ cups	REGULAR	1.50
CUPS, Weight, and Diameter Equivalents (page 61)		

Diet soda does not count towards your AIM (page 44) and moderation should be maintained. Limit intake to two a day and then de-caffeinated thereafter. If you do go over, it will not count toward your AIM.

Portion	Water [Ø]	CUPS
cup or more	WATER [Ø] including:	0
cup or more	.... Carbonated [Ø]	0
cup	.... Coconut*	0 or 1
* 1st CUP in a Day Does Not Count Towards Your AIM (page 44)		
cup or more	.... Flavored - low calorie [Ø]	0
cup or more	.... Mineral [Ø]	0
cup or more	.... Purified [Ø]	0
cup or more	.... Spring [Ø]	0
CUPS, Weight, and Diameter Equivalents (page 61)		

BREADS and GRAINS

Portion	Breads and Grains	CUPS
	BAGELS:	
small = 2 oz.	.... up to 3" (8cm) diameter	0.50
medium = 3 oz.	.... about 3" (8cm) diameter	0.75
	BREADS:	
1	.... Bread Slice, Biscuit, or Roll	0.50
1	.... Bun – burger or hot dog	1
cup = 4 oz.	.... Crumbs or Stuffing	1
	CEREALS:	
cup	.... Dry - low sugar preferred	1
cup (cooked)	.... Oatmeal - ½ cup uncooked	1
½ cup	CORNMEAL [Cx2] is ½ cup x2	1
½ cup	FLOUR [Cx2] is ½ cup x2	1
1	PANCAKE, 2-4" (5-10cm) diameter	0.50
cup (cooked)	PASTA - ½ cup uncooked	1
½ cup	+ Marinara Sauce [∅]	0
½ cup	+ Meat Sauce	0.50
½ cup	+ White Sauce [Cx2] is ½ cup x2	1
cup (cooked)	RICE – ½ cup uncooked	1
	TORTILLAS – corn or flour:	
small	.... 4.5" (11cm) diameter	0.25
medium	.... 6" (15cm) diameter	0.50
1	WAFFLE	0.50
CUPS, Weight, and Diameter Equivalents (page 61)		

DAIRY - Cheese and Creams

Portion	Cheese — LFP [Cx2]	CUPS
1 oz.	CHEESE DIP [Cx2] is ¼ cup x2	0.50
1 oz.	COTTAGE CHEESE [Cx2] is ¼ cup x2	0.50
1 oz.	CREAM CHEESE [Cx2] is ¼ cup x2	0.50
1 oz.	CURD type [Cx2] is ¼ cup x2	0.50
	.... Cheese Curds	
	.... Cottage or Ricotta	
1 oz.	GRATED CHEESE [Cx2] is ¼ cup x2	0.50
slice or 1 oz.	HARD CHEESE [Cx2] is ¼ cup x2	0.50
1 oz.	SHREDDED CHEESE [Cx2] is ¼ cup x2	0.50
slice or 1 oz.	SOFT CHEESE [Cx2] is ¼ cup x2	0.50
1 oz.	SPREAD [Cx2] is ¼ cup x2	0.50
CUPS, Weight, and Diameter Equivalents (page 61)		

Portion	Creams - LFP [Cx2]	CUPS
¼ cup or 4 tbsp.	COFFEE CREAMER[Cx2] is ¼ cup x2	0.50
¼ cup or 4 tbsp.	CREAM [Cx2] is ¼ cup x2	0.50
¼ cup or 4 tbsp.	EGGNOG [Cx2] is ¼ cup x2	0.50
¼ cup or 4 tbsp.	HALF & HALF [Cx2] is ¼ cup x2	0.50
¼ cup or 2 oz.	ICE CREAM [Cx2] is ¼ cup x2	0.50
¼ cup or 2 oz.	SOUR CREAM [Cx2] is ¼ cup x2	0.50
¼ cup or 2 oz.	WHIPPED CREAM [Cx2] is ¼ cup x2	0.50
¼ cup or 2 oz.	WHIPPING CREAM [Cx2] is ¼ cup x2	0.50
CUPS, Weight, and Diameter Equivalents (page 61)		

DAIRY – Eggs and Yogurt and Sweets

Portion	Eggs and Yogurt	CUPS
1	EGG - cooked any method:	0.25
2	.... Egg Whites - cooked	0.25
2	.... Egg Yolks – cooked	0.25
½ cup = 4 oz.	YOGURT - fat free preferred	0.50
1	3 EGG OMELET with Cheese	1.25
CUPS, Weight, and Diameter Equivalents (page 61)		

DESSERTS and SWEETS (1 of 2)

Portion	Desserts, Sweets [Cx2]	CUPS
small	BROWNIE [Cx2] is 1 cup x2	2
1/8 of 9" diameter	CAKE [Cx2] is 1 cup x2	2
6 pieces = 1 oz.	CANDY [Cx2] is ¼ cup x2	0.50
small	CANDY BAR [Cx2] is ½ cup x2	1
2 tbsp.	CARAMEL [Cx2] is ¼ cup x2	0.50
1 oz.	CHOCOLATE [Cx2] is ¼ cup x2	0.50
CUPS, Weight, and Diameter Equivalents (page 61)		

*Low calorie or low fat desserts and sweets are recommended. Many desserts and sweets are **Cx2** foods (page 65) and must be counted twice.*

Portion	Desserts and Sweets	CUPS
medium (3" diameter)	COOKIE [Cx2] is ½ cup x2	1
cup = 4 oz.	CRÈME BRÛLÉE [Cx2] is 1 cup x2	2
small	CUPCAKE [Cx2] is 1 cup x2	2
cup = 4 oz.	CUSTARD [Cx2] is 1 cup x2	2
small	DOUGHNUT [Cx2] is ½ cup x2	1
cup = 4 oz.	FLAN [Cx2] is 1 cup x2	2
2 tbsp.	FUDGE [Cx2] is ¼ cup x2	0.50
cup	GELATIN – low calorie preferred	1
cup	.... very very low calorie [∅]	0
cup = 4 oz.	ICE CREAM [Cx2] is 1 cup x2	2
1	PASTRY [Cx2] is 1 cup x2	2
1/8 of pie	PIE [Cx2] is 1 cup x2	2
cup = 4 oz.	PUDDING [Cx2] is 1 cup x2	2
cup	SORBET – low calorie preferred	1
cup	SOUFFLÉ – low calorie preferred	1
1	TART with fruit – low calorie preferred	1
cup = piece	TRES LECHE [Cx2] is 1 cup x2	2
CUPS, Weight, and Diameter Equivalents (page 61)		

*Low calorie or low fat desserts and sweets are recommended. Many desserts and sweets are **Cx2** foods (page 65) and must be counted twice.*

Portion	Burger King	CUPS
	BREAKFAST:	
1	.... Biscuit or Croissan'wich	2
	.... Breakfast Burritos:	
1	.... Sausage Burrito	1.50
½	.... Southwestern Burrito	1.50
1	.... Cinnabon [Cx2] is 1 cup x2	2
½	.... Double Croissan'wich	1.50
order	.... Kid's Oatmeal	1
1	.... Muffin with Egg & Cheese	1.50
order	+ Sausage or Ham	0.50
order	.... Oatmeal:	0.75
order	+ Maple & Brown Sugar	1.50
½ order	.... Pancake Sausage Platter	1.50
2 tbsp.	+ Syrup [Condiment] (page 79)	0.50
CUPS, Weight, and Diameter Equivalents (page 61)		

You can have up to a **COUPLE** *of* **CUPS** *per meal of any fast food. If it is over two cups, then reduce it to two cups or less. Following are cups approximations for specific fast foods. Reviewing these can also give a better understanding of how to estimate portions.*

Portion	Burger King	CUPS
	BREAKFAST cont.	
small order	.... Hash Brown [**Cx2**] is 1 cup **x2**	2
order	.... French Toast Sticks	0.50
¼	.... Ultimate Breakfast Platter	2
	DESSERTS:	
1	.... Dutch Apple [**Cx2**] is 1 cup **x2**	2
1	.... Ice Cream Cone [**Cx2**] is ¾ cup **x2**	1.50
1	.... Cookie [**Cx2**] is ½ cup **x2**	1
1	.... Ice Cream Cup [**Cx2**] is ¾ cup **x2**	1.50
1	.... Sundae [**Cx2**] is 1 cup **x2**	2
	SANDWICHES:	
1	.... BBQ Rib Sandwich	2
1	.... Big Fish:	2
½	.... Big Fish Deluxe	1.50
1	.... Cheeseburger:	1.50
1	.... Double Cheeseburger	2
½	.... Chicken Sandwich:	1.50
½	.... Crispy	1.75
1	.... Crispy or Grilled Chicken	2
1	.... Hamburger:	1
1	.... Double Hamburger	1.50
1	.... Turkey	2
CUPS, Weight, and Diameter Equivalents (page 61)		

Portion	Burger King	CUPS
	SANDWICHES cont.	
1	.... Veggie Burger	2
½	..... Whopper:	1.50
½	.... Double Whopper	2
1	.... Whopper Jr.	1.50
½	.... Whopper with Cheese	2
1	CHICKEN NUGGET [Cx2] is ¼ cup x2	0.50
2 pieces	CHICK'N STRIP [Cx2] is ½ cup x2	1
1	GARDEN or CEASAR SALADS	2
cup	MILKSHAKE [Cx2] is 1 cup x2	2
	SIDES:	
order	.... Apple Slices [FFF]	O
value order	.... French Fries [Cx2] is 1 cup x2	2
½ small order	.... French Fries [Cx2] is ¾ cup x2	1.50
½ medium order	.... French Fries [Cx2] is 1 cup x2	2
order	.... G & C Fries [Cx2] is 1 cup x2	2
1 stick	.... Cheese String [Cx2] is ¼ cup x2	0.50
value order	.... Onion Rings [Cx2] is ¾ cup x2	0.50
½ small order	.... Onion Rings [Cx2] is ¾ cup x2	1.50
½ medium order	.... Onion Rings [Cx2] is 1 cup x2	2
1	TACO	1
packet	TOPPINGS – all	0.50
CUPS, Weight, and Diameter Equivalents (page 61)		

Portion	Dairy Queen	CUPS
	BASKETS:	
½	.... Crispy Chicken Sandwich	1.50
1	.... Grilled Chicken Sandwich	1.50
order	.... Chicken Strip [Cx2] is 1 cup x2	2
	BURGERS:	
1	.... Homestyle Burger	1.50
slice or 1 oz.	+ Cheese [Cx2] is ¼ cup x2	0.50
½	.... California	1.50
	.... Cheeseburgers (CB):	
½	.... Homestyle Double CB	1.25
½	.... Bacon Double CB	1.50
½	.... Classic with Cheese	1.50
1	.... Grillburger	2
½	.... Mushroom Swiss	1.50
½	.... ¼ lb. Burgers - all	2
1	HOT DOG:	1
1	.... Chili Cheese Hot Dog	1.50
	SALADS:	
1	.... Crispy Chicken Salad	1.50
1	.... Grilled Chicken Salad	1
1	.... Side Salad [Ø]	0

CUPS, Weight, and Diameter Equivalents (page 61)

Portion	Dairy Queen	CUPS
	SIDES:	
½ small order	.... French Fries [Cx2] is ¾ cup x2	1.50
medium order	.... French Fries [Cx2] is 1 cup x2	2
½ order	.... Onion Rings [Cx2] is 1 cup x2	2
	ICE CREAM CONES:	
1	.... Dipped [Cx2] is 1 cup x2	2
1	.... Regular [Cx2] is 1 cup x2	2
1	.... Soft Serve [Cx2] is ¾ cup x2	1.50
	ROYAL TREATS:	
1	.... Blast [Cx2] is 1 cup x2	2
1	.... Parfait [Cx2] is 1 cup x2	2
	SUNDAES:	
1	.... small or ½ large [Cx2] is 1 cup x2	2
½	.... medium [Cx2] is ¾ cup x2	1.50
	NOVELTIES:	
1	.... Banana Split [Cx2] is 1 cup x2	2
1	.... Blizzard [Cx2] is 1 cup x2	2
½ slice	.... Blizzard Cake [Cx2] is 1 cup x2	2
1	.... DQ Sandwhich [Cx2] is 1 cup x2	2
	BEVERAGES:	
small	.... Artic Rush Slush	1
½ small	.... Malt or Shake [Cx2] is 1 cup x2	2
CUPS, Weight, and Diameter Equivalents (page 61)		

Portion	Kentucky Fried Chicken	CUPS
1 piece	BONELESS CHICKEN	1
	CRISPY CHICKEN - all types:	
1	.... Breast [M] & [Cx2] is 1 cup x2	2
1	.... Leg [M] & [Cx2] is ¾ cup x2	1.50
1	.... Thigh [M] & [Cx2] is 1 cup x2	2
1	.... Wing [M] & [Cx2] is ½ cup x2	1
	GRILLED CHICKEN [M]:	
1	.... Breast or Thigh [M]	1
1	.... Hot Wing [M]	0.50
1	.... Leg [M]	0.75
1	.... Wing [M]	0.50
1	CRISPY FILET [Cx2] is 1 cup x2	2
1	CRISPY STRIP [Cx2] is 1 cup x2	2
½	COUNTRY FRIED STEAK [Cx2] is 1 cup x2	2
	POPCORN CHICKEN:	
½ order	.... Individual Order [Cx2] is 1 cup x2	2
order	.... Original Bites [Cx2] ¼ cup x2	0.50
	SIDES:	
order	.... Baked Beans or Biscuit	1
order	.... Cole Slaw or Cornbread	1
1	.... Corn on the Cob, 3" (8cm)	0.50
CUPS, Weight, and Diameter Equivalents (page 61)		

Portion	Kentucky Fried Chicken	CUPS
	SIDES cont.	
order	.... Corn - sweet	0.50
order	.... Green Beans [∅]	0
order	.... Macaroni	1
	.... Potato:	
order	.... Mashed	0.50
order	.... Salad or Wedges	1
	DESSERTS:	
½ slice	.... Cake or Pie [Cx2] is 1 cup x2	2
1	.... Parfait [Cx2] is 1 cup x2	2
slice	.... Pie [Cx2] is 1 cup x2	2
1	.... Turnover [Cx2] is 1 cup x2	2
	OTHER:	
order	.... GoGo squeeze Applesauce	0.25
½ order	.... Country Fried Steak [Cx2] is 1 cup x2	2
order	.... Gizzards or Livers	1
order	.... Jalapeno Peppers [∅]	0
packet	.... Parmesan Garlic Croutons	0.25
1	.... String Cheese [Cx2] is ¼ cup x2	0.50
	POT PIES, BOWLS, BOXES:	
1	.... Chicken Pot Pie	2
CUPS, Weight, and Diameter Equivalents (page 61)		

Portion	Kentucky Fried Chicken	CUPS
	POT PIES, BOWLS, BOXES cont.	
½	.... Famous Bowl	2
½ value box	.... Popcorn Chicken	1.50
1	.... Snack Size Bowl	1
	SALADS:	
1	.... Caesar Salad	1.75
1	.... Caesar Side Salad	0.50
1	.... Crispy Chicken BLT	1.75
1	.... Side Salad [⊘]	0
	SALAD DRESSINGS:	
order	.... Buttermilk Ranch	0.75
order	.... Creamy Parmesan Caesar	1
order	.... Light Italian [⊘]	0
order	.... Ranch® Fat Free	0.25
	SANDWICHES:	
1	.... Chicken Littles	1.00
order	+ Sauce	0.50
1	.... Doublicious	2
1	.... Filet [Cx2] is 1 cup x2	2
1	.... Honey BBQ	1.50
1	.... Twister [Cx2] is 1 cup x2	2
order	+ Sauce	0.50

CUPS, Weight, and Diameter Equivalents (page 61)

FAST FOODS - McDonald's (1 of 2)

Portion	McDonald's	CUPS
	BREAKFAST:	
1	.... Bagel, Bacon, Cheese, Egg	2
½	.... Big Breakfast	2
1	.... Biscuit with Sausage	2
1	+ Egg	0.25
1	.... Egg McMuffin or Burrito	1.50
1	.... Egg White McMuffin	1
order	.... Fruit and Maple Oatmeal	1.50
1	.... Hash Brown [Cx2] is ½ cup x2	1
1	.... Hotcake or Cinnamon Melt	2
½ order	.... Hotcakes and Sausage	1.50
1	.... McGriddle	2
1	.... McMuffin without Egg	2
½	.... Steak, Egg, Cheese Bagel	1.75
	BURGERS & SANDWICHES:	
½	.... Bacon Clubhouse Burger	2
½	.... Big Mac	1.50
1	.... Cheeseburger	1.50
1	.... Hamburger	1
1	.... McDouble	2
1	.... Premium Crispy Club	1.50
½	.... ¼ Pounder with Cheese	2

CUPS, Weight, and Diameter Equivalents (page 61)

Portion	McDonald's	CUPS
	CHICKEN:	
1	.... McNugget [Cx2] is ¼ cup x2	0.50
1	FRUIT 'n YOGURT PARFAIT	1.50
	McCAFE:	
small	.... Frape Mocha	2
small	.... Iced Coffee or Latte	0.75
small	.... Mocha	1.50
	SALADS:	
1	.... Caesar or Ranch	0.50
1	.... Fruit and Walnut	1
1	.... Side Salad [Ø]	0
1	.... Southwest Chicken:	1.50
½	.... Southwest Crispy Chicken	1.25
1	.... Southwest Grilled Chicken	2
	SIDES:	
order	.... Apple Dippers	0.25
small order	.... French Fries [Cx2] is ¾ cup x2	1.50
medium order	.... French Fries [Cx2] is 1 cup x2	2
½ large order	.... French Fries [Cx2] is ¾ cup x2	1.50
	SNACK WRAPS:	
½	.... Crispy Chicken - all	1.50
1	.... Grilled Sweet Chili Chicken	1.50
CUPS, Weight, and Diameter Equivalents (page 61)		

135

Portion	Panda Express	CUPS
	APPETIZERS:	
1	.... Chicken Egg Roll	0.75
1	.... Rangoon [Cx2] is ½ cup x2	1
1	.... Crispy Shrimp [Cx2] ¼ cup x2	0.50
order	.... Hot and Sour Soup	1
1	.... Potsticker	1
1	.... Veggie Spring Roll	0.75
	BEEF ENTREES:	
order	.... Beijing, Broccoli, Shanghai	2
	CHICKEN ENTREES:	
order	.... Black Pepper	1
order	.... Grilled Teriyaki	1.50
order	.... Kung Pao Chicken	1
order	.... Mushroom Chicken	0.75
order	.... Orange or Sweetfire	2
order	.... Shitake Kale Breast	0.75
order	.... String Bean Breast	0.75
	DESSERTS:	
1	.... Choc. Cookie [Cx2] ½ cup x2	1
1	.... Fortune Cookie [Cx2] ¼ cup x2	0.50
order	EGGPLANT TOFU	1
order	MIXED VEGETABLES [∅]	0
CUPS, Weight, and Diameter Equivalents (page 61)		

Portion	Panda Express	CUPS
order	PORK - all entrees	2
	SAUCES:	
packet	.... Chili Sauce	0
packet	.... Hot Mustard [∅]	0
packet	.... Mandarin	0
packet	.... Plum or Potsticker	0
packet	.... Soy Sauce [∅]	0
packet	.... Sweet and Sour	1.50
packet	.... Teriyaki	0.75
	SEAFOOD:	
order	.... Golden Szechuan	1.50
	.... Shrimp:	
1	.... Crispy [Cx2] is ¼ cup x2	0.50
order	.... Golden Treasure	2
order	.... Honey Walnut	2
	SIDES:	
order	.... Chow Mein	2
order	.... Rice:	2
order	.... Brown or White	2
order	.... Fried Rice	2
1	SOBE GREEN TEA	2
1	SOBE LEAN BEVERAGE [∅]	0
CUPS, Weight, and Diameter Equivalents (page 61)		

FAST FOODS - Pizza Hut

Portion	Pizza Hut	CUPS
order	BREAD or BREADSTICK	1
	BUFFALO WINGS:	
2 wings	.... Garlic	1
2 wings	.... Medium	1
	DESSERTS:	1
slice	.... Apple or Cherry Pizza	1
1	.... Cinnamon Stick	0.50
order	.... White Icing [Cx2] is ½ cup x2	1
	PASTAS:	
order	.... Cavatini or Lasagna	2
1	P'ZONE - all types	2
	PIZZA:	
slice	.... Meat Lovers	1
slice	.... Cheese Crust Pepperoni	2
	.... Personal Pan:	
½ pizza	.... Meat Lovers	2
½ pizza	.... Veggie Lovers	1.75
slice	.... Stuffed Crust	2
slice	.... Veggies Lovers Thin	1
slice	.... 12" (30cm)	1
slice	.... 14" (35cm)	2
CUPS, Weight, and Diameter Equivalents (page 61)		

138

FAST FOODS - Subway

Portion	Subway	CUPS
order	BREAD	1
1	BREAKFAST SANDWICH	1
1	COOKIE [Cx2] is 1 cup x2	2
1	FLATBREAD	1
	SALADS:	
1	.... Black Ham or Turkey	0.50
1	.... Chicken Teriyaki - all types	1
1	.... Club or Roast Beef	0.75
1	.... Oven Roasted Chicken	0.75
1	.... Veggie Delight	0.25
	SANDWICHES:	
1	.... BLT	1.50
1	.... Italian BMT	2
1	.... Mini Sub - all types	0.75
1	.... Smokehouse BBQ	2
1	.... 6" Chicken Melt	2
1	.... 6" Subs - all types	1
	SOUPS:	
order	.... Chicken Noodle or Tomato	0.50
order	.... Chili	2
order	.... Clam Chowder	1
CUPS, Weight, and Diameter Equivalents (page 61)		

Portion	Taco Bell	CUPS
1	EMPANADA - all types [Cx2] is 1 cup x2	2
1	BURRITOS - are all 2 cups, except:	2
1	.... Bacon and Egg	1
½	.... Cantina	2
1	.... Sausage and Egg	0.50
½	.... XXL Grilled Stuffed	2
1	CHALUPA	1.50
	FRESCOS:	
1	.... Burrito Supreme	1
1	.... Chicken, Crunchy or Steak	0.75
	GORDITAS:	
1	.... Cheesy Gordita Crunch	2
1	.... Gordita Supreme	1.50
	SIDES:	
order	.... Beans or Latin Rice	0.50
order	.... Chips and Corn Salsa	1
order	.... Chips and Guacamole	1.50
1	.... Churro or Cinnamon Twist	1
1	.... Cookie Sandwich	2
order	.... Fiesta Potatoes	1.50
order	.... Pintos and Cheese	1
CUPS, Weight, and Diameter Equivalents (page 61)		

Portion	Taco Bell	CUPS
	NACHOS:	
½ order	.... BellGrande	2
order	.... Cheesy Nachos	1
order	.... Nachos Supreme	2
½ order	.... Volcano	2
	SPECIALTIES:	
½	.... AM Crunchwraps	2
1	.... Griller or Quesadilla	2
½	.... Cantina Bowl	1.50
1	.... Cheese Roll-Up	1
1	.... Crunchwrap Supreme	2
1	.... Enchirito	1.50
½	.... Mexican Pizza	1.50
1	.... MexiMelt	1
	TACO SALADS:	
½	.... Express Salad with Chips	1.50
½	.... Fiesta Salad	2
	TACOS - crunchy or soft:	
1	.... Beef, Supreme, Volcano	1
1	.... Chicken or Fresco - all types	0.75
1	.... Doritos Locos or Steak	1
CUPS, Weight, and Diameter Equivalents (page 61)		

Portion	Wendy's	CUPS
large order	CHILI	2
	CRISPY CHICKEN NUGGET:	
1	.... Nugget [Cx2] is ¼ cup x2	0.50
packet	DRESSING - all	0.50
	FRIES - natural cut:	
½ order	.... small [Cx2] is ¾ cup x2	1.50
½ order	.... medium [Cx2] is 1 cup x2	2
¼ order	.... large [Cx2] ½ cup x2	1
	KID'S MEALS:	
1	+ Cheeseburger	1.50
1	+ Hamburger	1
	SANDWICHES:	
½	.... Asiago Ranch Club:	2
½	.... Homestyle Chicken	1.50
½	.... Spicy Chicken	2
¼	... Baconator:	1
¼	.... Son of Baconator	2
1	.... Cheddarburger	2
1	.... Double Stack	2
1	.... Hamburger	1
1	.... Jr. Bacon Cheeseburger	2
CUPS, Weight, and Diameter Equivalents (page 61)		

Portion	Wendy's	CUPS
	SANDWICHES cont.	
1	.... Jr. Cheeseburger	1.50
1	.... Jr. Cheeseburger Deluxe	2
½	.... ¼ lb. Single	1.50
½	.... ½ lb. Double	2
¼	.... ¾ lb. Triple	1
	.... Chicken Sandwiches:	
1	.... Crispy Chicken	2
½	.... Homestyle Chicken	1.50
1	.... Monterey Chicken	2
½	.... Spicy Chicken Fillet	1.50
1	.... Ultimate Chicken Grill	2
	SIDES:	
order	.... Apple Slices [**FFF**]	0
order	.... Baked Potato	1.25
order	+ Sour Cream and Chives	0.25
order	.... Buttery Spread with Cracker	0.50
1	.... Caesar Chicken Go	1
1	.... Caesar Side Salad	0.25
1	.... Garden Side Salad [Ø]	0
packet	SWEET and SOUR SAUCE	0.25
1	WENDY'S FROSTY	2
CUPS, Weight, and Diameter Equivalents (page 61)		

FAST FOODS - White Castle
and Wingstop

Portion	White Castle	CUPS
1	BREAKFAST SANDWICHES	1.50
	BURGERS:	
1	.... Dbl. Bacon Cheeseburger	2
1	.... White Castle Burger	0.75
order	+ Cheese or Bacon	0.50
3	CHICKEN RINGS	1
1	FISH with CHEESE	1
3	MOZZARELLA CHEESE STICKS	1
1	SURF and TURF	2
CUPS, Weight, and Diameter Equivalents (page 61)		

Portion	Wingstop	CUPS
order	BOURBON BAKED BEANS	1
order	CREAMY COLE SLAW	0.75
3	CRISPY VEGGIE STICKS [Ø]	0
order	DIPS or SAUCES	0.50
order	FRESH CUT SEASONED FRIES	2
order	POTATO SALAD	0.75
2	WINGS - all types	0.50
CUPS, Weight, and Diameter Equivalents (page 61)		

Below is a sampling of "Fresh Fruits". Their Spanish / French / Italian translations may follow as well as their AKA (also known as).

Up to two cups of any fresh fruit in a single day will not count towards your **AIM** *(noted as the 0 under the CUPS column). Beyond two cups will count cup for cup (noted as 1). For example, if you had a mango and an apple AND a banana, then you would count the banana as one cup (noted as the 1 under the CUPS column).*

In other words you will have to count all "Fresh Fruits" after your first two cups in a day. You cannot carry over uneaten cups of fresh fruit to the next day.

Fresh Fruits – ¼ each [FFF]	CUPS
BREADFRUIT / *Buen Pan* / *Arbre à Pain*	O or 1
CHERIMOYA (chirimoya or custard apple)	O or 1
COCONUT / *Coco* / *Noix de Coco*	O or 1
DURIAN (king of fruits)	O or 1
MELON - all types / *Melón* / *Melon* / *Melone*	O or 1
PINEAPPLE / *Piña* / *Ananas* / *Anana*	O or 1
SAPOTE / *Zapote* / *Sapote* / *Sapota*	O or 1
SOURSOP / *Guanabana* / *Corossol*	O or 1

In the table that is above are some specific "Fresh Fruits", all of which ¼ of that specific "Fresh Fruit" will equal a one cup portion and depending on how much you have in a day will determine whether you have to count it towards your daily food intake, that is, your **AIM** (**A**djusted **I**ndividual **M**easurement).

Remember that your 1st two fresh fruits in a day do not count as they are from the [**FFF**] *Special Food Category.*

Fresh Fruits - 1 each [FFF]	CUPS
APPLE / *Manzana / Pomme / Mela*	O or 1
AVOCADO / *Aguacate / Avocat / Avocado*	O or 1
BANANA / *Banana / Banane / Banana*	O or 1
BLOOD ORANGE (anti-aging orange)	O or 1
GRAPEFRUIT / *Toronja / Pamplemousse*	O or 1
MANGO / *Mango / Mangue / Mango*	O or 1
MOMBIN (jobo or Spanish plum)	O or 1
NASEBERRY (mamey or zapote)	O or 1
ORANGE / *Naranja / Orange / Arancione*	O or 1
ORANGELO / *Chironja*	O or 1
PAPAYA / *Lechosa / Papaye / Papaia*	O or 1
PEACH / *Durazno / Pêche / Pesca*	O or 1
PEAR / *Pera / Poire / Pera*	O or 1
POMEGRANATE / *Granada / Granade*	O or 1
POMELO (lusho fruit)	O or 1

In the table above are "Fresh Fruits", of which ¼ of the "Fresh Fruit" equals a one cup portion and depending on how much of this "Fresh Fruit" you have in a day will determine whether you have to count it towards your **AIM** (page 44).

Fresh Fruits - 2 each [FFF]	CUPS
APRICOT / *Albaricoque* / *Abricot* / *Albicocca*	O or 1
CLEMENTINE / *Naranja Clemintina*	O or 1
FEIJOA (guavasteen or pineapple guava)	O or 1
GUAVA / *Guayaba* / *Goyave* / *Guaiava*	O or 1
HICACO / *Icaco* (coco plum)	O or 1
KIWIFRUIT (Chinese gooseberry or kiwi)	O or 1
LEMON / *Limón* / *Citron* / *Limone*	O or 1
LIME / *Limón Verde* / *Citron Vert* / *Limetta*	O or 1
MANDARIN ORANGE (mandarine)	O or 1
NECTARINE (smoothed skinned peach)	O or 1
PASSION FRUIT / *Chinola or Maracuya or Parcha*	O or 1
PERSIMMON / *Caqui* / *Kaki* / *Caco*	O or 1
PITAYA FRUIT (dragon fruit or pithaya)	O or 1
PLUM / *Ciruela* / *Prune* / *Prugna*	O or 1
SATSUMA ORANGE (mandarin or mikan)	O or 1
STARFRUIT / *Carambola* / *Carambole*	O or 1
TANGERINE / *Tangerina* / *Mandarine*	O or 1
QUINCE (fruit of love)	O or 1

In this table are "Fresh Fruits", of which two equals a one cup portion and depending on how much you have in a day will determine whether it counts.

Fresh Fruits - 1 cup [FFF]	CUPS
ACKEE (akee or achee or ackee apple)	0 or 1
BERRIES - all types / *Baya / Baie / Bacca*	0 or 1
CHERRY / *Cereza / Cerise / Ciliegia*	0 or 1
CURRANT – black or red or white	0 or 1
DATE / *Dátil / Datte / Dattero*	0 or 1
FIG / *Higo / Figue / Fico*	0 or 1
GRAPE - all types / *Uva / Raisin / Uvetta*	0 or 1
JACKFRUIT (jaca or jack or jakfruit)	0 or 1
JAMUN FRUIT (black plum or jambo)	0 or 1
KUMQUAT / *Quinoto / Kumquat*	0 or 1
LYCHEE / *Lichi / Litchi / Lichee*	0 or 1
OLIVES - all types / *Oliva / Olive / Oiliva*	0 or 1
PEEWAH (peach palm or pejibaye)	0 or 1
RAMBUTAN / *Mamón Chino / Ramboutan*	0 or 1
STRAWBERRY / *Fresa / Fraise / Fragola*	0 or 1
TAMARIND FRUIT / *Tamarindo / Tamarin*	0 or 1

In the table above table are "Fresh Fruits", of which one of the "Fresh Fruit" equals a one cup portion and depending on how much you have in a day will determine whether it count it towards your **AIM** *(page 44).*

FRUITS (non-fresh) and PRODUCTS

Portion	Fruits and Products	CUPS
4 oz.	APPLESAUCE – low calorie preferred	0.50
1 oz.	CANDIED FRUIT [Cx2] ¼ cup x2	0.50
½ can	CANNED FRUIT - all types	0.50
½ cup	DRIED FRUIT – low calorie preferred	0.50
½ cup	FROZEN FRUIT - all types	0.50
½	FRUIT BREAKFAST BAR	0.50
5	FRUIT CHEWS [Cx2] ¼ cup x2	0.50
½ cup	FRUIT JELL-O – low calorie preferred	0.50
½ cup	FRUIT JUICE - all types	0.50
2	FRUIT ROLL-UP	0.50
½ cup = 4 oz.	YOGURT - fat free preferred	0.50
1 oz.	GLAZED FRUITS	0.50
2 tbsp.	JAM [Condiment] (page 79)	0.50
2 tbsp.	JELLY [Condiment]	0.50
2 boxes = 1½ oz.	RAISINS (about 20)	0.50
CUPS, Weight, and Diameter Equivalents (page 61)		

Include fruit at every meal (fresh if at all possible) and in snacks. Frozen fruit, canned fruit, fruit juices, and fruit products will always count toward your daily food intake, that is, your AIM *(page 44).*

Portion	Meat - all types [M]	CUPS
slice **CTS** ¼ cup	BACON - all types, lean preferred	0.25
4 oz. **CTS** 1 cup	BEEF - all cuts, lean preferred:	1
slice **CTS** ¼ cup	.... Roast Beef	0.25
4 oz. **CTS** 1 cup	BRATWURST - lean preferred	1
	CHICKEN – skinless preferred:	
4 oz. **CTS** 1 cup	.... Baked, Grilled or Roasted	1
4 oz. **CTS** 1 cup	.... Breast	1
3 oz. **CTS** ¾ cup	.... Leg	0.75
3 oz. **CTS** ¾ cup	.... Thigh	0.75
2 oz. **CTS** ½ cup	.... Wing	0.50
slice **CTS** ¼ cup	COLD CUTS – lean preferred	0.25
4 oz. **CTS** 1 cup	DUCK – skinless preferred	1
CUPS, Weight, and Diameter Equivalents (page 61)		

The cup approximation for all meats is based upon a 4 oz. (113g) portion. This 4 oz. portion of any meat product will count as one cup towards your AIM *(page 44). Remember that 4 oz. counts (**CTS**) 1 cup, 2 oz. **CTS** ½ cup and 1 oz. **CTS** ¼ cup.*

Portion	Meat - all types [M]	CUPS
4 oz. **CTS** 1 cup	FISH or SEAFOOD - all types	1
4 oz. **CTS** 1 cup	GOAT – lean preferred	1
2 oz. **CTS** ½ cup	HOT DOG – lean preferred	0.50
4 oz. **CTS** 1 cup	PORK – lean preferred:	1
slice **CTS** ¼ cup	.... Ham	¼
4 oz. **CTS** 1 cup	POULTRY - includes canned:	1
1 oz. **CTS** ¼ cup	.... Gizzards	0.25
1 oz. **CTS** ¼ cup	.... Livers	0.25
2 oz. **CTS** ½ cup	SAUSAGE - lean preferred	0.50
4 oz. **CTS** 1 cup	SHEEP – lean preferred:	1
4 oz. **CTS** 1 cup	.... Lamb or Mutton	1
	SHELLFISH:	
4 oz. **CTS** 1 cup	.... Baked or Grilled or Steamed	1
6 small or 1 oz.	.... Clam	¼
4 oz. **CTS** 1 cup	.... Lobster	1
1 or 1 oz.	.... Oyster - shucked	¼
4 oz. **CTS** 1 cup	.... Shrimp:	1
	25 small, 20 medium, 5 large, 2 jumbo	
CUPS, Weight, and Diameter Equivalents (page 61)		

Crispy, battered, or fried meats are **Cx2** food (page 65) and as a result their CUPS amount in the right column must be doubled.

NUTS and SEEDS

Portion	Nuts and Seeds [Cx2]	CUPS
¼ cup	NUTS & SEEDS [Cx2] is ¼ x2	0.50
¼ cup = 25	.... Almonds [Cx2] is ¼ cup x2	0.50
¼ cup = 5	.... Brazil Nuts [Cx2] is ¼ cup x2	0.50
¼ cup = 20	.... Cashews [Cx2] is ¼ cup x2	0.50
¼ cup = 5	.... Chestnuts [Cx2] is ¼ cup x2	0.50
¼ cup = 25	.... Hazelnuts [Cx2] is ¼ cup x2	0.50
¼ cup = 25	.... Hickory [Cx2] is ¼ cup x2	0.50
¼ cup = 10	.... Macadamia [Cx2] is ¼ cup x2	0.50
¼ cup = 30	.... Peanuts [Cx2] is ¼ cup x2	0.50
¼ cup = 15	.... Pecans [Cx2] is ¼ cup x2	0.50
¼ cup = 200	.... Pine Nuts [Cx2] is ¼ cup x2	0.50
¼ cup = 15	.... Pistachios [Cx2] is ¼ cup x2	0.50
¼ cup = 15	.... Walnuts [Cx2] is ¼ cup x2	0.50
¼ cup = 1 oz.	MIXED NUTS [Cx2] is ¼ cup x2	0.50
CUPS, Weight, and Diameter Equivalents (page 61)		

Because of their nutritional composition, all nuts and seeds must be counted twice when determining food intake throughout. As an aid in remembering foods in this category, recall that Count begins with "C" and that Cashews also begin with "C".

PIZZA

Portion	Pizza	CUPS
	FROZEN:	
slice	.... DiGiorno 200 calorie slice	1
¼ pizza	.... Jack's Original Pepperoni	1.50
order	.... Lea. Cuisine French Bread	1.50
¼ pizza	.... Red Baron Four Cheese	1
¼ pizza	.... 12" (30cm) Tombstone	1.50
¼ pizza	.... 12" Totino Crispy Party Pizza	1
¼ pizza	.... Stonefire Thin Vegetable	1
	REGULAR THICKNESS PIZZA:	
slice	.... round, 1/8 of a pizza	1.50
slice	.... square, 4" x 4" (5cm x 5cm)	1.50
½ small	PAN PIZZA	2
	THICK PIZZA:	
½ slice	.... large 16" (40cm)	1
slice	.... round, 1/8 of a pizza	2
slice	.... square, 4" x 4" (5cm x 5cm)	2
slice	THIN PIZZA	1
CUPS, Weight, and Diameter Equivalents (page 61)		

You can have a **COUPLE** of **CUPS** a day (1-2 slices) depending upon size and thickness. Your hand may represent a slice (1½ cups).

SANDWICHES

When making a sandwich, count each slice of bread as ½ cup, for a total of 1 cup. If you add a thin slice of cheese (¼ cup) count it twice because it is a **Cx2** food. A thin slice (1 oz.) of meat counts (**CTS**) as ¼ cup, and now you have a total of 1¾ cups. You need not count any vegetables such as, lettuce, onions, pickles, tomatoes, etc., and you may not need to count the condiment(s) used in the sandwich (see "CONDIMENT PRODUCTS", page 79).

SNACK FOODS (Chips)

You can estimate chips in a number of ways. A small bag (1 oz.) counts 1 cup and is the equivalent of 10 chips, EXCEPT for fat free low calorie chips. Snack examples follow.

Portion	SNACKS (½ cup)	CUPS
small = 2 oz.	BAGEL, up to 3" (8cm) diameter	0.50
Slice	BREAD – whole wheat preferred	0.50
2	BR. RICE CAKES – low salt	0.50
1	CARROTT [Ø]	O
¼ cup	+ Hummus [Cx2] is ¼ cup x2	0.50
2 sticks	CELERY [Ø]	O
2 slices	+ wrapped with Ham	0.50
slice = 1 oz.	CHEESE – LFP [Cx2] is ¼ cup x2	0.50
10 oz.	CHIPS, small bag – LFP	0.50
½ cup	CINNAMON PUFFS	0.50
¼ cup = 1 oz.	COTTAGE CHEESE [Cx2] is ¼ cup x2	0.50
10	CRACKERS – whole grain	0.50
2 oz. CTS ½ cup	+ Tuna [M]	0.50
½ small bar	CHOCOLATE [Cx2] is ¼ cup x2	0.50
2	EGGS – cooked any method	0.50
½ cup	FIGS [FFF]	O
any amount	+ Cinnamon & Mint	O
1 oz. = 2 tbsp.	+ Mascarpone Cheese [Cx2] is ¼ cup x2	0.50
½ cup	FRUIT JUICE or SMOOTHIE	0.50
½	GRANOLA or LUNA BAR	0.50
2 oz. CTS ½ cup	JERKY - all types [M]	0.50
CUPS, Weight, and Diameter Equivalents (page 61)		

Portion	SNACKS (½ cup)	CUPS
¼ cup	NUTS or SEEDS [Cx2] is ¼ cup x2	0.50
½ cup cooked	OATMEAL – ¼ cup uncooked	0.50
mini-bag	POPCORN – LFP	0.50
1	POPSICLE	0.50
½	PROTEIN BAR – LFP	0.50
½ cup = 4 oz.	PUDDING – LFP	0.50
small box	RAISINS	0.50
2 packages	SALMON JERKY	0.50
½	SHRIMP SPRING ROLL	0.50
½ cup	SOUP	0.50
1 = 1 oz.	STRING CHEESE [Cx2] is ¼ cup x2	0.50
3 slices	TOMATO with OLIVE OIL [Condiment]	0
1 oz.	+ Feta Cheese [Cx2] is ¼ cup x2	0.50
½ medium	TORTILLA	0.50
small carton	VANILLA SOY MILK	0.50
2 tbsp.	WHITE BEAN DIP	0.50
	+ NO Count Vegetables [Ø]	0
10	WHOLE GRAIN CRACKER and BASIL	0.50
¼ cup = 1 oz.	+ Goat Cheese [Cx2] is ¼ cup x2	0.50
½ cup = 4 oz.	YOGURT - fat free preferred	0.50
1	100 CALORIE SNACK PACK	0.50
CUPS, Weight, and Diameter Equivalents (page 61)		

Vegetables [∅]	CUP$
ARTICHOKES / *Alcachofa* / *Artichut*	o
ARUGULA (garden rocket or roquette)	o
ASPARAGUS / *Aspárrago* / *Asperge*	o
BAMBOO SHOOTS / *Telón de Bambú*	o
BEAN SPROUTS / *Brotes de Soja*	o
BEETS (blood turnip or garden/red beet)	o
BOK CHOY (Chinese or flowering cabbage)	o
BROCCOFLOWER (green cauliflower)	o
BROCCOLI / *Brócoli* / *Brocol* / *Broccoli*	o
BROCCOLI RABE (raab or turnip broccoli)	o
BRUSSELS SPROUTS / *Coles de Bruselas*	o
CABBAGE / *Repollo* / *Chou* / *Cavolo*	o
CAIGUA (lady's slipper or slipper gourd)	o
CARROTS / *Zanahoria* / *Carotte* / *Carota*	o
CAULIFLOWER / *Coliflor* / *Choufluer* / *Cavolfiore*	o

This is a sampling of the "**NO** count vegetables".

Spanish / French / Italian translations may follow and AKA (also known as). If it is a vegetable and not in these tables and not a "**C/C** vegetable", *you do not have to count these veregtables towards your* AIM *(page 44).*

Vegetables [∅]	CUPS
CELERIAC (celery root or knob celery)	o
CELERY / *Apio / Céleri / Sedano*	o
CHARD (silver or spinach beet)	o
CHRISTOPHENE / *Tayota or Chayote / Mirliton*	o
CHICORY (succor or blue dandelion)	o
COLLARD GREENS / *Berza / Chou Cavalier*	o
CUCUMBERS - inc. pickles / *Pepino*	o
EGGPLANT / *Berenjena / Aubergine*	o
ENDIVE / *Endibia / Endive / Indivia*	o
GARDEN CRESS (cress or land cress)	o
GARLIC / *Ajo / Ail / Aglio*	o
GREEN (French) BEANS / *Ejotes or Vainitas*	o
JICAMA / *Castano* (Mexican water chestnut)	o
KALE (flowering cabbage)	o
KOHLRABI (German or cabbage turnip)	o
LEEKS / *Puerro / Poireau / Porro*	o
LETTUCE / *Lechuga / Laitue / Latuga*	o
MUSHROOMS / *Hongo / Champignon / Fungo*	o
MUSTARD GREENS (Indian mustard)	o
OKRA / *Guingombó or Molondron / Gombo*	o
ONIONS / *Cebolla / Oignon / Cipolla*	o
OPUNTIA (paddle cactus or prickly pear)	o

Vegetables [Ø]	CUPS
PARSNIP / *Chirivía* / *Panias* / *Pastinaca*	O
PEAS / *Guisantes* / *Pois* / *Piselli*	O
PEPPER - all types and is a fruit but counts as vegetable / *Aji*	O
PUMPKIN - all types	O
RADICCHIO / *Achicoria Roja* / *Trévis*	O
RADISHES / *Rábano* / *Radis* / *Ravanello*	O
RHUBARB / *Ruibarbo* / *Rhubarbe* / *Rabarbaro*	O
RUTABAGA (Swede or Swedish turnip)	O
SCALLION / *Cebollin* (green or spring onion)	O
SEAWEED / *Alga* / *Algues* / *Alghe*	O
SHALLOT / *Chalote* / *Échalotte* / *Scalogno*	O
SORREL (narrow leaf dock or spinach dock)	O
SPINACH / *Espinaca* / *Épinards* / *Spinaci*	O
SQUASH - all types / *Calabazas*	O
TOMATILLO – a fruit but counts as vegetable	O
TOMATO - a fruit but counts as vegetable	O
TURNIPS / *Nabo* / *Navet* / *Rapa*	O
WATER CHESTNUT (Ling or Singhara nut)	O
WATERCRESS / *Berro* / *Cresson* / *Crescione*	O
ZUCCHINI / *Calabacín* / *Courgette* / *Zucchino*	O

*These are all **NO** count [Ø] Vegetables.*

VEGETABLES [C/C]

Portion	Vegetables [C/C]	CUPS
	C = **C**ORN [C/C]:	
1	.... Corn on the Cob - 3" (8cm) [C/C]	0.5
cup	.... Sweet Corn [C/C]	1
	U = LEGUMES [C/C]:	
cup	.... Beans [C/C] except green beans	1
cup	.... Black Eye Peas [C/C]	1
cup	.... Chickpeas [C/C]	1
cup	.... Lentils [C/C]	1
cup	.... Tofu [C/C]	1
	P = **P**OTATOES [C/C]:	
¾ cup = 4 oz.	.... Au Gratin Potatoes [C/C]	0.75
	.... Baked Potato [C/C]:	
small	.... 1-2" diameter or < 8 oz.	0.50
medium	.... 2-3" (5-8cm) diameter or 8 oz.	1
large	.... > 3" (8cm) diameter or > 8 oz.	1.50
cup	.... Fried [C/C] [Cx2] is 1 cup **x2**	2
cup	.... Mashed Potatoes [C/C]	1
¾ cup = 4 oz.	.... Potato Salad [C/C]	0.75
cup	.... Plantains [C/C]	1
cup	.... Sweet Potatoes [C/C]	1
cup	.... Yams [C/C] or Yuca [C/C]	1
CUPS, Weight, and Diameter Equivalents (page 61)		

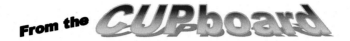

MASCARO FAMILY RECIPES

Next are recipes from the **CUP**board. These are **Mascaro Family** favorites.

These recipes provide some very simple illustrations of how to determine CUP amounts from actual recipes. This helps to demonstrate that you can enjoy ALL of your favorite foods and recipes and still lose weight on **the CUPS diet®**.

All of these recipes can be reduced proportionally. The CUP amount for each portion has already considered any SPECIAL FOOD CATEGORIES instructions.

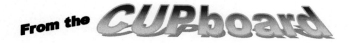

From the CUPboard

MASCARO FAMILY RECIPES

Boursin Stuffed Mushrooms – Matt Mascaro
Bread (no-knead) – Patty Mascaro
Caesar Salad – Joe Mascaro
Chicken Pot Pie – Angie Mascaro
Crab Cakes – Matt Mascaro
Crusted Pork Chops – Andrea Greer (Mascaro)
Double Pie Crust – Angie Mascaro
Flan – Dr. Hilda Mascaro
Grilled Pita Pizza – Dr. Jimmy Mascaro
Italian Roasted Potatoes – Angelo Mascaro
Mediterranean Potato Salad – Joe Mascaro
Morir Soñando– Dr. Hilda Mascaro
Salsa – Dr. Jimmy Mascaro
Spinach Dip – Andrea Greer (Mascaro)
Taco Rico – Patty Mascaro

BOURSIN STUFFED MUSHROOMS
by Matt Mascaro

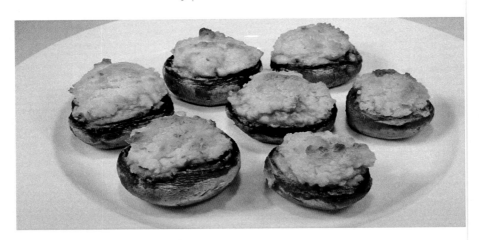

To enlarge all photographs,
double tap photo (on many devices).

Portion	Stuffed Mushrooms	CUPS
¼ cup = 1 oz.	CREAM CHEESE [Cx2] is ¼ cup x2	0.50
½ cup = 2 oz.	BOURSIN CHEESE [Cx2] is ½ cup x2	1
¼ cup	PANKO BREAD CRUMBS	0.25
14-16 = 8 oz.	BUTTON MUSHROOMS [∅]	0
sprinkle	KOSHER SALT [∅]	0
	Total CUPS in Recipe	**1.75**

DIRECTIONS

- **Cheese (Boursin and cream cheese)**
  ..... warm cheese to room temperature
  ..... in a bowl mix cheese together
  ..... add ¼ cup of Panko bread crumbs
  ..... use enough to hold mixture together
- **Mushrooms**
  ..... remove mushroom stems & discard
  ..... spoon or pipe filling into mushrooms
  ..... fill where stem used to be & above
  ..... place mushrooms on a baking sheet
- **Bake 20-25 minutes at 425°F (218°C)**
  ..... cheese should turn golden brown
  ..... very lightly sprinkle with Kosher salt

CUPS AMOUNT
Total countable cups in recipe = 1.75
1.75 cups / 14-16 mushrooms = 0.125
2 mushrooms x 0.125 x 2 = 0.50 cup
EXAMPLE: 2 mushrooms count ¼ cup

BREAD
4th generation "no knead" recipe
by Patty Mascaro

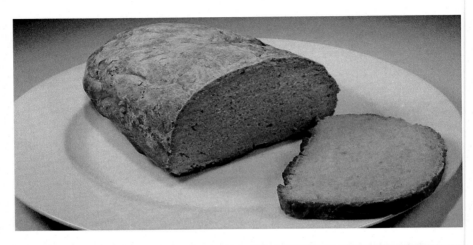

Portion	Bread "no knead"	CUPS
¾ cup	MILK	0.75
tsp.	CRISCO SHORTENING [**Condiment**]	O
¼ cup	SUGAR [**Cx2**] is ¼ cup **x2**	0.50
1¼ tsp.	SALT [**Ø**]	O
½ cup	WATER [**Ø**] added to the milk	O
¼ cup	WATER [**Ø**] for the yeast	O
½ tsp.	REGULAR RISE YEAST [**Ø**]	O
3½ cups	FLOUR [**Cx2**] is 3½ cups **x2**	7
tsp.	BUTTER [**Condiment**]	O
	Total CUPS in Recipe	**8.25**

DIRECTIONS

- **Milk based mixture**
  ..... scald milk, add shortening & sugar
  ..... add ½ cup of warm water with salt
- **Yeast and water mixture**
  ..... put yeast in ¼ cup of warm water
  ..... let yeast & water proof (bubble)
  ..... add yeast mixture to milk & flour
  ..... well work dough into a ball
- **Cover dough with greased plastic wrap**
  ..... allow to rise until it doubles in size
  ..... you can divide dough into 2-3 loaves
  ..... place loaves on a greased pan
  ..... cover loaves once again
  ..... let loaves rise till they double in size
- **Bake 50-60 minutes at 350°F (177°C)**
  ..... then brush tops with melted butter

CUPS AMOUNT
EXAMPLE: slice counts ½ cup

CAESAR SALAD
by Joe Mascaro

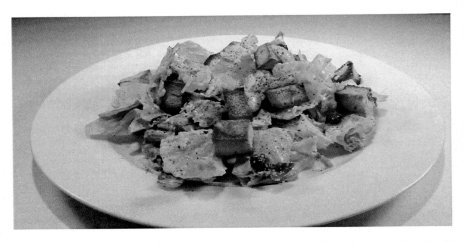

Portion	Caesar Salad Dressing	CUPS
tsp.	1. GREY POUPON DIJON MUSTARD [Ø]	O
1½ tsp.	2. RED WINE VINEGAR [Ø]	O
2 tsp.	3. WORCESTERSHIRE SAUCE [Ø]	O
1	4. EGG	0.25
2 oz. **CTS** ½ cup	5. ANCHOVY FILLETS - in oil [**M**]	0.50
3–4 cloves	6. minced GARLIC [Ø]	O
cup = 10 oz.	PARMESAN **C**HEESE [**Cx2**] is 1 cup **x2**	2
cup	extra virgin OLIVE OIL [**Cx2**] is 1 cup **x2**	2
½-1 tsp.	fresh squeezed LEMON JUICE [Ø]	O
tsp. of each	BLACK PEPPER [Ø] & salted CAPERS [Ø]	O
1	HEART of ROMAINE LETTUCE [Ø]	O
	Total CUPS in Recipe	**4.75**

DIRECTIONS

- **Blend ingredients 1 to 6**
  ..... then slowly add 2 cups of parmesan
- **SLOWLY blend in oil in a small stream**
  ..... add to rinsed heart of romaine lettuce
  ..... toss with ¼ cup of grated parmesan
  ..... add lemon juice & fresh black pepper
  ..... garnish with fine salted Sicilian capers
- **Add croutons or toasted bread**
  ..... may use store bought
  ..... may use homemade (no-knead bread)
- **Because of raw egg, eat within 3 days**

CUPS AMOUNT
1 tsp. dressing does not count*
>1 tsp. counts a minimum of ½ cup*
*see Chapter 11 (Oils/Fats)
Over ¼ cup portions are counted twice
 see Chapter 9 (Cx2** food type)
EXAMPLE: ¼ cup dressing counts ½ cups

CHICKEN POT PIE
by Angie Mascaro

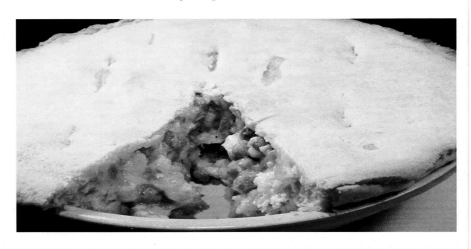

Portion	Chicken Pot Pie	CUPS
1	DOUBLE PIE CRUST – recipe found on page 176	7
1 lb. **CTS** 4 cups	skinless CHICKEN BREAST [**M**]	4
cup of each	CARROTS [**Ø**] & frozen PEAS [**Ø**]	O
medium	cubed POTATO (page 161) - 2-3" diameter [**C/C**]	1
½ cup of each	diced CELERY [**Ø**] & ONION [**Ø**]	O
½ cup = 1 stick	BUTTER [**Cx2**] is ½ cup **x2**	1
½ cup	FLOUR [**Cx2**] is ½ cup **x2**	1
½ tsp.	SALT [**Ø**]	O
¼ tsp. of each	BLACK PEPPER [**Ø**] & CELERY SEED [**Ø**]	O
2 cups	CHICKEN BROTH [**Ø**]	O
cup	MILK	1
	Total CUPS in Recipe	**15**

DIRECTIONS

- **Make "Double Pie Crust Pastry" (recipe)**
- **Put cubed chicken in water in large pot**
  ..... add sliced carrots, potatoes & celery
  ..... cover, boil 10 minutes, add peas, boil 5 minutes
  ..... drain very well, cover & set it aside
- **Melt butter in saucepan (medium heat)**
  ..... sauté diced onion until they are tender
  ..... whisk flour, salt, pepper, & celery seed
  ..... whisk in broth & milk for 1 minute
  ..... simmer & stir until thick for 10 minutes
- **Line deep pie dish with bottom pie crust**
  ..... add chicken, vegetables, & then sauce
  ..... cover with top crust (with slits cut in)
  ..... bake 45-50 minutes at 400°F (204°C)

CUPS AMOUNT
15 countable cups / 8 slices = 1.875
1.875 cups rounds up to 2 cups
EXAMPLE: 1/8 slice of pie counts 2 cups

CRAB CAKES
by Matt Mascaro

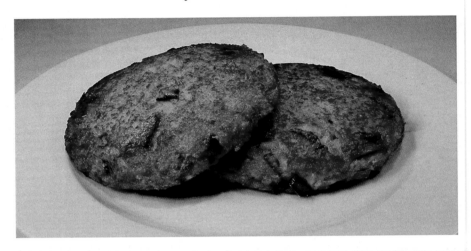

Portion	Crab Cakes	CUPS
2	EGGS	0.50
¼ cup	MAYONNAISE [**Cx2**] is ¼ cup **x2**	0.50
¼ cup	diced RED ONION [**Ø**]	0
¼ cup	diced RED PEPPER [**Ø**]	0
½ cup	diced GREEN PEPPER [**Ø**]	0
tbsp.	OLD BAY SEASONING [**Ø**]	0
¾ lb. **CTS** 3 cups	LUMP CRAB MEAT [**M**]	3
tsp.	WORCESTERSHIRE SAUCE [**Ø**]	0
tsp.	HOT SAUCE [**Ø**] is optional	0
1¼ cups	PANKO BREAD CRUMBS	1.25
¼ cup = ½ stick	clarified BUTTER [**Cx2**] is ¼ cup **x2**	0.50
	Total CUPS in Recipe	**5.75**

DIRECTIONS

- **Crab cakes**
  - ..... whisk eggs & mayonnaise
  - ..... add seasonings, onions, & peppers
  - ..... add lump crab meat
  - ..... lightly mix ingredients
  - ..... slowly add 1 cup Panko bread crumbs
  - ..... use enough crumbs to form 6 wet balls
  - ..... coat outside with ¼ cup bread crumbs
- **Preheat oven to 425°F (218°C)**
- **Sauté crab cakes in clarified butter**
  - ..... brown cakes on one side & then flip
- **Place in Oven 10-15 Minutes**
- **Serve with favorite sauce**

CUPS AMOUNT
Total countable cups in recipe = 5.75
5.75 cups / 6 crab cakes = 0.958
0.958 cups rounds up to 1 cup
EXAMPLE: 1 crab cake counts 1 cup

CRUSTED PORK CHOPS
by Andrea Greer (Mascaro)

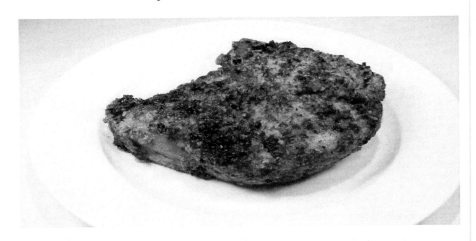

Portion	Crusted Pork Chops	CUPS
¾ cup	FRENCH'S FRIED ONIONS [**Cx2**] is ¾ cup **x2**	1.50
10	butter flavored CRACKERS	0.50
tbsp.	MRS. DASH SEASONING BLEND [**Ø**]	0
2	EGGS	0.50
20 oz. **CT$** 5 cups	4 boneless PORK CHOPS [**M**]	5
¼ tsp.	SALT [**Ø**]	0
¼ cup = ½ stick	BUTTER or OIL [**Cx2**] is ¼ cup **x2**	0.50
¼ tsp.	fresh ground BLACK PEPPER [**Ø**]	0
	Total CUP$ in Recipe	8

DIRECTIONS

- **Crusting mixture**
    ..... crush fried onions in shallow bowl
    ..... add crackers & crush with onions
    ..... add seasoning blend
- **Whip eggs in 2nd bowl**
    ..... coat pork chops with egg
    ..... cover pork chops with breading mix
- **Frying pan (medium heat)**
    ..... use butter or oil (optional)
    ..... brown pork chops & turn over
    ..... salt & pepper as desired
- **Place in baking pan in oven**
    ..... bake at 350°F (177°C) for 45-50 minutes

CUPS AMOUNT
Total countable cups in recipe = 8
8 cups / 4 boneless pork chops = 2
This is a **Cx2** food (**C**ount times **2**)
EXAMPLE: 1 pork chop counts 2 cups

DOUBLE PIE CRUST
by Angie Mascaro

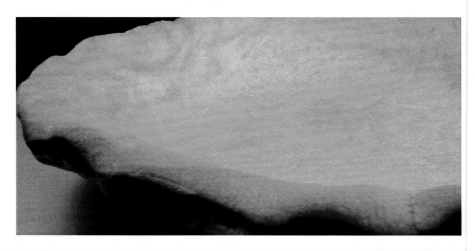

Portion	Double Pie Crust	CUPS
This is for "2" pie crusts (top & bottom) and can be used for Chicken Pot Pie		
2½ cups	FLOUR [**Cx2**] is 2½ cups **x2**	5
½ tsp.	SALT [**Ø**]	O
½ cup	SHORTENING [**Cx2**] is ½ cup **x2**	1
½ cup = stick	cubed BUTTER [**Cx2**] is ½ cup **x2**	1
cup	ICE WATER [**Ø**]	O
	Total CUPS in Recipe	**7**

DIRECTIONS

- **This is for "two" pie crusts (top & bottom)**
  ..... for Chicken Pot Pie recipe
  ..... for bottom only, cut recipe in half
- **Mix flour & salt together**
  ..... "cut in" chilled butter flavor shortening
  ..... "cut in" chilled cubed butter till crumbly
  .... mix & rub pieces between fingers
  .... it should resemble coarse oatmeal
- **Add up to ½ cup of ice water**
  ..... toss with fork until it comes together
  ..... add additional ice water as needed
- **Form ball & chill 30 minutes**
  ..... divide in half & roll out for 2 pie crusts

CUPS AMOUNT
Total countable cups in recipe = 7
EXAMPLE: 3½ cups for a single pie crust
EXAMPLE: 7 cups for a double pie crust*
*Used in the Chicken Pot Pie recipe

FLAN
by Dr. Hilda Mascaro

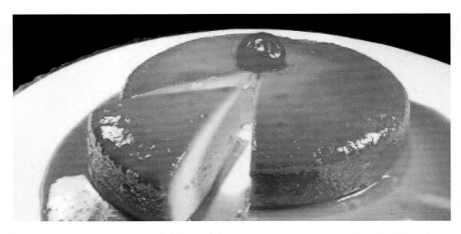

Portion	Flan	CUPS
cup	WHITE SUGAR [**Cx2**] is 1 cup **x2**	2
4	EGGS	1
	CANNED MILK:	
1¼ cups	..... Condensed Milk [**Cx2**] is 1¼ cups **x2**	2.50
1½ cups	..... Evaporated Milk [**Cx2**] is 1½ cups **x2**	3
	OPTIONAL GARNISH	
slice	+ Pineapple [**FFF**]	0
1	+ Cherry [**FFF**]	0
	Total CUPS in Recipe	**8.5**

DIRECTIONS

- **Melt sugar in flan mold (medium saucepan)**
  ..... caramelize sugar over medium heat
  ..... allow caramel to darken (do not burn)
  ..... swirl caramel over sides of mold
  ..... let mold cool & caramel harden
  ..... start hot water bath in large pot (with lid)
- **Custard mixture**
  ..... beat eggs in bowl
  ..... add condensed milk & evaporated milk
  ..... put mixture in mold, then in water bath
  ..... gently boil 50-60 minutes with lids on
  ..... boil till it sets (knife comes out clean)
- **Remove flan mold from water bath & chill**
  ..... invert mold, pour caramel over flan

CUPS AMOUNT
Total countable cups in recipe = 8.50
8.50 cups / 8 portions = 1.0625 & round up
EXAMPLE: 1/8 slice counts as 1¼ cups

GRILLED PITA BREAD PIZZA
by Dr. Jimmy Mascaro

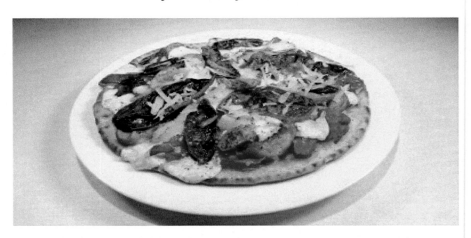

Portion	Grilled Pita Bread Pizza	CUPS
1	PITA FLAT BREAD	1
tsp.	OLIVE OIL [**Condiment**]	O
¼ cup	TOMATOES with roasted GARLIC [**Ø**]	O
2 tbsp.	chopped ONION [**Ø**]	O
4 leafs	fresh BASIL [**Ø**]	O
¼ cup = 1 oz.	fresh MOZZARELLA [**Cx2**] is ¼ cup **x2**	0.50
¼ cup = 1 oz.	MOZZARELLA [**Cx2**] is ¼ cup **x2**	0.50
sprinkle	KOSHER SALT [**Ø**]	O
clove	diced GARLIC [**Ø**]	O
½ tsp.	OREGANO [**Ø**]	O
¼ cup = 2 oz.	sliced MUSHROOMS [**Ø**] optional	O
	Total CUPS in Recipe	**2**

DIRECTIONS

- **Set barbecue to medium temperature**
- **Pita bread**
  - ..... brush or spray bottom with olive oil
  - ..... brush or spray top with olive oil
- **Toppings**
  - ..... mushrooms, onions, peppers, etc.
  - ..... shredded mozzarella
  - ..... pieces of sliced fresh mozzarella
- **Lower heat to medium-low**
  - ..... cook 4-7 minutes till cheese has melted
- **Remove from BBQ & add fresh basil**
  - ..... spray lightly with olive oil
  - ..... place on BBQ for up to 1 minute
  - ..... sprinkle a tiny pinch of salt over top

CUPS AMOUNT
Total countable cups in recipe = 2
2 cups / 4 slices = 0.50 cup
EXAMPLE: slice counts as ½ cup

ITALIAN ROASTED POTATOES
by Angelo Mascaro

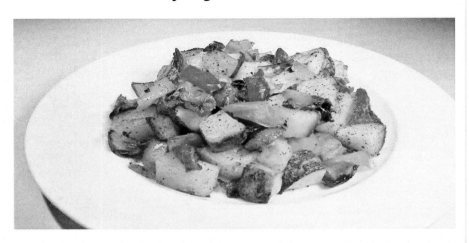

Portion	Roasted Potatoes	CUPS
6 cups = 2 lbs.	POTATOES (page 161) - cubed [C/C]	6
½ cup	sliced medium ONION [∅]	O
¼ cup	OLIVE OIL [Cx2] is ¼ cup x2	0.50
1	chopped GREEN PEPPER [∅]	O
1	chopped RED PEPPER [∅]	O
½ tsp.	fresh ground BLACK PEPPER [∅]	O
¾ tsp.	SALT [∅]	O
3-4	chopped fresh MINT LEAVES [∅]	O
4 cloves	minced GARLIC [∅]	O
	Total CUPS in Recipe	**6.50**

DIRECTIONS

- **Potatoes**
  - ..... scrub & wash potatoes
  - ..... peeling potatoes is optional
  - ..... slice & cube potatoes (bite size)
  - ..... place in a casserole type pan
- **Add to potatoes**
  - ..... onions (sliced)
  - ..... peppers (cut into bite size squares)
  - ..... garlic cloves (minced)
  - ..... fresh mint leaves
  - ..... fresh ground black pepper
- **Heat 40-60 minutes at 375-400°F (204°C)**
  - ..... stir & turn vegetables often
  - ..... cook till they are slightly crusted
  - ..... salt lightly before serving

CUPS AMOUNT
All portions will count cup for cup
EXAMPLE: 1 cup portion counts 1 cup

MEDITERRANEAN POTATO SALAD
by Joe Mascaro

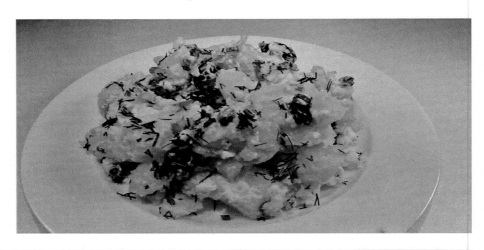

Portion	Potato Salad	CUPS
6 cups = 2 lbs.	RUSSET POTATOES (page 161) - cubed [**C/C**]	6
2 tbsp.	fresh squeezed LEMON JUICE [**FFF**]	O
2 tbsp.	OLIVE OIL (**Condiment**)	0.50
½ cup = 4 oz.	plain GREEK YOGURT - LFP	0.50
tsp. of each	SUGAR [**Condiment**] & SEA SALT [**Ø**]	O
½ tsp.	fresh ground BLACK PEPPER [**Ø**]	O
4	chopped SCALLIONS [**Ø**]	O
2 tbsp.	CAPERS - without vinegar [**Ø**]	O
20	KALAMATA OLIVES - in wine sauce [**Ø**]	O
cup = 6 oz.	FETA CHEESE [**Cx2**] is 1 cup **x2**	2
2 tbsp.	finely chopped DILL WEED [**Ø**]	O
	Total CUPS in Recipe	9

DIRECTIONS

- **Potatoes**
  - ..... peel, then cube (bite size) potatoes
  - ..... boil until "almost" done, drain, **cool**
- **Lemon juice mixture**
  - ..... dissolve sugar in lemon juice
  - ..... add olive oil & **Greek** yogurt
  - ..... add sea salt & ground black pepper
- **Place potatoes in large bowl**
  - ..... add sliced scallions
  - ..... slowly mix in capers & feta cheese
  - ..... add sliced **Kalamata** olives
  - ..... pour yogurt mix over top, gently mix
- **Top potato salad**
  - ..... with chopped dill weed
  - ..... may add additional crumbled feta

CUPS AMOUNT
All portions will count cup for cup
EXAMPLE: 1 cup portion counts 1 cup

MORIR SOÑANDO

"to die dreaming"

by Dr. Hilda Mascaro

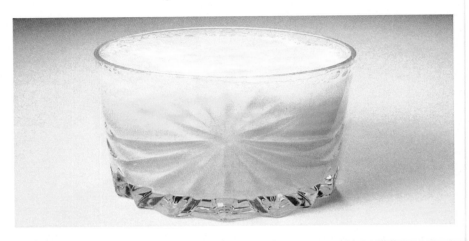

Portion	Morir Soñando [Cx2]	CUPS
1½ cups	EVAPORATED MILK [**Cx2**] is 1½ cups **x2**	3
¼ cup	SUGAR [**Cx2**] is ¼ cup **x2**	0.50
½ cup	MILK	0.50
2 cups	ORANGE JUICE	2
2 cups	ICE CUBES [**∅**]	0
	Total CUPS in Recipe	6

DIRECTIONS

- **Dilute sugar in evaporated milk**
  ..... add milk to the above mixture
  ..... then add 2-3 cups of ice
  ..... stir & chill **very**, **very**, **very** well
  ..... now add orange juice & mix well
- **Makes 4 one cup servings (with ice)**

Morir Soñando is a very popular and unique drink of the Dominican Republic, and has been around for generations. It literally translates "to die dreaming." Usually served as a mid-afternoon snack or a dinner drink, but Morir Soñando can be enjoyed any time of the day.

CUPS AMOUNT
This is a **Cx2** food (page 65) item
EXAMPLE: 1 cup (without ice) counts 2 cups
EXAMPLE: 1 cup (with ice) counts as 1 cup

SALSA
by Dr. Jimmy Mascaro

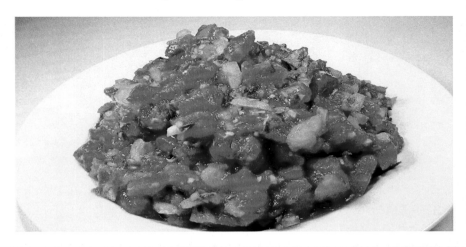

Portion	Salsa	CUPS
14.5 oz. (411g)	petit diced TOMATOES [⊘]	o
14.5 oz. (411g)	diced TOMATOES with mild GREEN CHILES [⊘]	o
tbsp.	fresh squeezed LIME JUICE [⊘]	o
2 tsp.	minced GARLIC [⊘]	o
tbsp.	chopped mild GREEN CHILES [⊘]	o
tsp.	SALT [⊘]	o
small	diced ONION [⊘]	o
½ cup	finely chopped CILANTRO [⊘]	o
	OPTIONAL INGREDIENTS:	
½ cup	..... Mango [**FFF**] or Hot Pepper [⊘]	o
Total CUPS in Recipe		⊙

DIRECTIONS

- **Combine cans of diced tomatoes**
  ..... add salt, garlic, onions, & cilantro
  ..... add chopped mild green chiles
  ..... add fresh squeezed fresh lime
  ..... mix above (do not put in a blender)
- **Chill for 1 hour**
- **Drain liquid before serving**
- **Optional ingredients**
  ..... ½ chopped roasted arbol pepper (chopped)
  ..... ½ cup of diced mango
  ..... ½ cup of finely diced green pepper
  ..... ½ cup of sweet corn
  ..... add additional lime juice if desired
- **May use as a Taco Rico Recipe topping**

CUPS AMOUNT
This is a **NO** count recipe food item*
*Chapter 9, page 63 (Vegetables)
EXAMPLE: Any portion size will not count [Ø]

SPINACH DIP
by Andrea Greer (Mascaro)

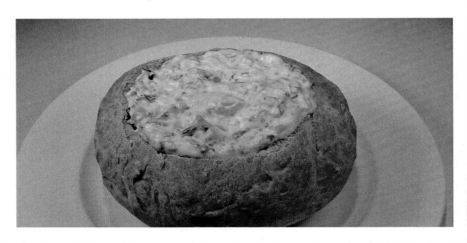

Portion	Spinach Dip [Cx2]	CUPS
packet	dried VEGETABLE SALAD MIX [∅]	O
10 oz.	chopped frozen SPINACH [∅]	O
2 cups	MAYONNAISE [Cx2] is 2 cups x2	4
2 cups	SOUR CREAM [Cx2] is 2 cups x2	4
8 oz.	chopped WATER CHESTNUTS [∅]	O
	OPTIONAL INGREDIENTS:	
¼ cup	..... diced Onions [∅]	O
4-8 oz.	..... chopped Artichoke Hearts [∅]	O
2-3	..... diced Green Onions [∅]	O
clove	..... minced Garlic [∅]	O
	Total CUPS in Recipe	8

DIRECTIONS

- **Thaw & drain the frozen spinach**
- **Spinach dip mixture**
    ..... combine sour cream & mayonnaise
    ..... mix in dried vegetable salad mix
    ..... add diced water chestnuts & spinach
    ..... stir & mix very well
- **Chill for 1 hour before serving**
- **Serve with**
    ..... crackers, bread, or a bread bowl
    ..... bread (no-knead Bread recipe)
    ..... add cup amounts for crackers or bread

CUPS AMOUNT
1 tsp. does not count*
>1 tsp. counts a minimum of ½ cup*
*see Chapter 11, page 79 (Condiments/Creams)
¼ cup portions or more are counted twice
 see Chapter 9, page 63 (Cx2** food type)
EXAMPLE: ¼ cup counts as ½ cup

TACO RICO
by Patty Mascaro

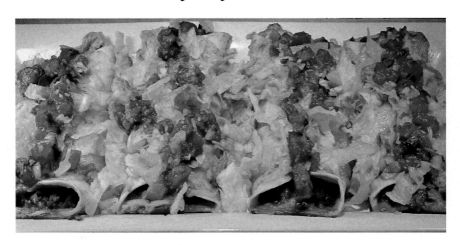

Portion	Taco Rico	CUPS
1¼ cups	CREAM of CHICKEN SOUP	1.25
1¼ cups	can of MILK – use the above soup can	1.25
1¼ cups of each	CHICKEN BROTH [Ø] & WATER [Ø]	O
tsp. of each	OREGANO [Ø] & minced GARLIC [Ø]	O
1 lb. **CTS** 4 cups	ground BEEF - LFP [M]	4
tsp. of each	SALT [Ø] & SAGE [Ø] & CUMIN [Ø]	O
½ tbsp.	CHILI POWDER [Ø]	O
tbsp.	chopped mild GREEN CHILES [Ø]	O
½ cup	chopped ONION [Ø]	O
6	medium flour TORTILLAS	3
½ cup = 2 oz.	**C**HEDDAR **C**HEESE [**Cx2**] is ½ cup **x2**	1
	Total CUPS in Recipe	**10.50**

DIRECTIONS

- **Sauce (use soup can to measure liquids)**
  - ..... mix soup, water, milk, broth, & oregano
  - ..... add sage, cumin, & simmer 30 minutes
- **Ground beef**
  - ..... brown, add garlic, chili powder, & chiles
  - ..... add sautéed onions & half of the sauce
- **Flour tortillas**
  - ..... place tortillas on a greased cookie sheet
  - ..... fill each tortilla with up to ½ cup of beef
  - ..... close tortillas & top with ¼ cup of sauce
  - ..... sprinkle the tops with cheddar cheese
- **Cover & bake 25 minutes at 350°F (177°C)**
- **Uncover & bake for 5 more minutes**
- **Top with lettuce, tomatoes, or salsa (page 188)**

CUPS AMOUNT
10.5 countable cups / 6 Taco Ricos = 1.75
EXAMPLE: 1 Taco Rico counts 1¾ cups

FINAL COMMENTS

From Dr. MASCARO

If you have questions, comments, or suggestions email drmascaro@thecupsdiet.com or visit www.thecupsdiet.com and select "contact" in the upper right corner and send a message. I want your experience with **the CUPS diet®** *to be a positive one and to work for you. So .... let ME work for you and help with motivation and encouragement as well as addressing your specific progress.*

the CUPS diet® *has a user support forum on FACEBOOK. Please select* **the CUPS diet®** *page, "'Like" it and you will have access to discuss user motivation, weight loss tips, weight loss results, nutrition, and exercise. The forum can also be used to find out the opinions of others, as well as for asking questions, conducting a poll, or simply keeping in touch with other users.*

A Spanish version will soon be available, and look for **KUPS for KIDS™**, *a new weight management method, based on* **the CUPS diet®**.

INDEX

About Dr. Mascaro, 16, 17, 163
Ackee, 149
Advantages of the eBook, 20
AIM - Adjusted Individual Measurement
    22, 23, 42-50, 52-56, 63-65, 67-71,
    73-75, 79, 80, 82, 86, 90, 117, 119-
    121, 145-147, 149-151, 158
Allows for Dining Out, 28, 60
Allows for Easy Meal Planning, 28
Almonds and Nuts, 153
Am. Society for Nutritional Science, 71
Amazon.com, 18
American Diabetes Association, 17
American Medical Association, 17
American Psychiatric Association, 17
American Society for Nutrition, 17
An Actual User's Progress Tracking, 54
Anchovy, 168
Android, 19, 21
Anorexia Nervosa, 26
Anxiety, 27
Apples, 64, 68, 76, 96, 128, 135, 145, 147
Applesauce, 132, 150
Apricot, 148
Artichokes, 150, 190
Artificial Sweetener, 70, 97, 119
Arugula, 158
Asparagus, 158
Assns., Societies, Organizations, 17
Atherosclerosis, 30
Average Size Fist (volume estimator), 57
Avocado, 147
Baba Ghanoush, 81
Bacon, 144, 151
Bagel, 72, 76, 91, 122, 134, 156
Baked Beans (legUmes), 131, 144
Baking Powder or Soda, 70
Bamboo Shoots, 160
Banana, 146
Barley Malt Syrup, 81
Baseball (volume estimator), 57
BBQ Sauce, 80

bDesign Photography, 14
Bean Sprouts, 158
Beans (legUmes), 65, 67, 161
Beef, 62, 69, 77, 110, 136, 139, 141, 151,
    192, 193
Beer, 118
Beets, 81, 158
Behavior, 26, 27, 30
Belief, 49
Berries, 149
Biking, 89
Biscuit, 122, 126, 131, 134
Bite of Food (volume estimator), 57
Black Eye Peas (legUmes), 161
Blood Orange, 147
Blood Sugar, 5
Blueberries, 72, 76, 91, 93, 149
BMI - Body Mass Index, 22, 23, 31-33,
    36, 38, 51
BMI Online Calculator, 31
BMR - Basal Metabolic Rate, 22, 23, 31
    42, 44, 46, 48, 52, 75, 85-89
Body Builders and Composition, 31, 36
Body Mass, 87, 89
Body Surface Area, 87
Body Temperature, 22, 43, 87, 88
Bok Choy, 158
Book Access, 23, 46, 50
Boursin Stuffed Mushrooms (recipe), 164
Bratwurst, 151
Brazil Nuts, 153
Bread, 57, 62-65, 69, 95, 122, 131, 138,
    139, 154-156, 163, 166, 167, 171, 182
    Crumbs, 122, 164, 172, 173
    No-knead (recipe), 163, 166, 167
Breadfruit, 146
Breakfast, 71, 72, 74, 76, 82, 127, 134,
    139, 144, 150
Breakfast Burrito, 126, 134
Breakfast Examples, 90-97
Breast-Feeding, 31, 36

Broccoflower, 158
Broccoli, 8, 76, 98, 136, 158
Broccoli Rabe, 158
Brown Rice Syrup, 81
Brown Sugar, 81, 126
Brussells Sprounts, 158
Bun (hamburger or hot dog), 122
Burgers, 126-129, 134, 142-144
Burrito, 103, 126, 134, 140, 195
Butter, 62, 66, 76, 80, 81, 143, 166, 167, 168, 170-177
C/C - **C**UP for **C**UP Vegetables, 23, 63, 65, 67, 70, 75, 76, 90, 98, 108, 117, 158, 161, 170, 182, 184
Cabbage, 158
Caesar Salad, 133, 163, 168, 169
Caiuga, 158
Cake, 66, 124-126, 130
Calcium, 8, 64
Caloric Deprivation, 86
Caloric Restrictions, 89
Calories, 8, 22, 28, 42, 43, 47, 64, 85
Can of Soda (volume estimator), 57
Cancer, 30, 33, 34
Candied or Glazed Fruits, 150
Candy, 66, 124
Cane Sugar, 81
Canola Oil, 80
Capers, 70, 81, 168, 169, 184, 185
Caramel, 66, 81, 119, 124, 179
Cardiac Rehab, 6
Carrots, 76, 156, 158, 170, 171
Cauliflower, 158
Celeriac, 159
Celery, 156, 159, 170, 171
Cell Phone (volume estimator), 57
Chard, 159
Chayote (christophen), 159
Cheese, 8, 63, 64, 66, 72, 80, 81, 91, 96, 97, 106, 108, 109, 117, 123, 124, 126-129, 132, 134, 138, 140-144, 154-157, 164, 165, 168, 181, 184, 185, 192, 193
Cheeseburger, 117, 127, 134, 142-144
Cherimoya, 146

Cherries, 149
Chestnuts and Nuts, 153
Chicory, 159
Chickpeas (leg**U**mes), 65, 67, 161
Chicken, 62, 69, 70, 76, 98, 105, 127, 129, 131-133, 135, 136, 139, 140-144, 151, 163, 170, 171, 192, 193
    Nuggets, 128, 135, 142
    Pot Pie (recipe), 170, 171, 176
    Sandwich, 127, 129, 133, 143
    Strips, 128, 129, 131
    Wings, 138, 144
Chili, 77, 129, 135, 137, 142
Chips, 140, 155, 156
Chocolate, 66, 81, 124, 156
Chocolate Syrup, 81
Christophene, 159
Chronic Disease, 30
Chronically Ill, 31, 36
Cilantro, 77, 188, 189
Clams, 139, 152
Clementines, 148
Coconut, 146
Coffee, 57, 70, 72, 76, 123
    Café Latte, Cappuccino, Mocha, 119
Coffee **C**reamer, 80
Coffee Mug (volume estimator), 57
Cole Slaw, 131, 144
Collards or Collard Greens, 159
Companion Website, 18, 24, 37, 44, 45, 49, 51-56, 78, 85
Competitive Athletes, 31, 36
Condensed Milk, 66, 80, 120, 178, 179
Condiments, 64, 70, 76, 77, 79-81, 106
Continue, 50, 51
Control **U**sing **P**ortion**S**™, 22, 30, 42
Cookie, 66, 125, 127, 136, 139, 140
Corn, 67, 132, 140, 161
    Oil, 80
    On the Cob, 131
    Sugar, 81
Cornmeal, 67, 122
Cortisol, 88
Cottonseed Oil, 80

Count Begins with the Letter "**C**", 66, 153
COUPLE of CUPS, 23, 63, 69, 82, 117, 126, 154
Crab Cakes (recipe), 163, 172, 173
Crackers, 62, 64, 104, 143, 156, 157, 174
Cravings, 7
Cream, 66, 72, 79, 80, 119, 123, 191
Croutons, 63, 132, 169
Crusted Pork Chops (recipe), 174, 175
Cucumbers, 159
CUPS Approximation (photo), 62
Cupcake, 66, 125
Currants, 149
Cx2 - **C**ount times **2**, 22, 64-67, 69, 70, 79, 117, 124, 125, 152, 155, 169, 175
Daily Menu "SAMPLE", 74, 76-78,
Dairy Products, 63, 64, 66, 71, 79, 80-82
Dairy Spread, 81
Date of Birth (age), 9, 23, 85
Dates, 149
Deck of Cards (volume estimator), 57
Degree of Muscularity, 31, 36
Dept. of Health & Human Services & Dept. of Agriculture, 89
Department of Psychology at the University of Texas In El Paso, 71
Depression, 27
Des Moines University, 16, 17
Desired Weight, 23, 35, 37
Development of **the CUPS diet**®, 25-29
Diabetes, 30, 33, 34
Diet, 39, 40
Diet Soda, 70, 121
Dietary Guidelines for Americans '05, 89
Dietary Restrictions, 86
Diets Low in Iodine, 86
Dinner, 55, 71, 74, 77, 90, 187
Dinner Examples, 90, 104-110
Dinner Roll, 122
Dipping Sauce, 80
Disease Risks Based on **BMI**, 33
Doctor of Osteopathic Medicine, 17
Does Not Require Supplements, 28
Dominican Medical Assn., Inc., 17

Double Pie Crust (recipe), 163, 170, 171
Doughnut, 66, 125
Dr. Hilda M. Mascaro, 14, 16, 163, 178
Dr. Jimmy R. Mascaro, 16, 17, 163
drmascaro@thecupsdiet.com, 19, 194
Duck, 151
Durian, 146
Dyslipidemia, 33
Easy to Follow in the Long-Term, 28
Eating Disorders Unit, 26
eBook, 1-4, 18-20, 45, 195
Book Access, 23, 46, 50
Egg, 57, 62, 64, 66, 72, 76, 92, 124, 126, 128, 134, 140, 156, 168, 169, 172
Eggnog (**C**hristmas), 66, 123
Eggplant (aubegine), 159
Emotional Issues, 27
Endive, 159
ENJOY your Favorite Foods, 8, 28, 29, 41, 83, 84, 162
Enter CUPS by the Day or the Meal, 52
Epinephrine, 88
Estimating CUPS (portion/food volume), 22, 26, 40, 57
Estimating Large Portions, 59
Evaporated Milk, 66, 80, 120, 178, 179, 186, 187
Examples of Healthy Meals, 78, 90
Examples of User's **AIM** Amounts, 47
Excessive Weight Loss, 86
Exercise, 5, 6, 19, 42, 48, 83, 89, 194
External Temperature, 87, 88
Extreme (crash) Dieting, 86
Extreme Fluid Loss, 87
Extreme Obesity, 31
FACEBOOK, 19, 196
Fad Diets, 15, 39, 40
Family-Friendly, 28
Fast Foods, 126-144
Fat (adipose) Tissue, 86
Fat Free, 64, 79, 95, 111, 112, 127, 155
FEAR (health consequence), 35, 37
Feta **C**heese, 157, 184, 185
Figs, 149

FFF - First Fruits Free, 23, 64, 65, 67, 70, 72, 75-77, 83, 90, 91, 93-97, 104, 108, 115, 117, 128, 143, 146-149, 156, 178
Fiber, 64
Finger (volume estimator), 57
Fish Sandwich, 127, 144
Flan, 66, 125 (recipe), 163, 178, 179
Fleischbutter, 81
Flour, 65, 67, 122, 166, 167, 170, 176
Food Approximations in CUPS, 117-161
Food Diaries, 71, 86
Food Groups, 23, 39, 63, 65, 69, 82
Food Restrictions, 5, 26, 27, 39
Food Volume, 22, 26, 40, 57-59
Forum on FACEBOOK, 19, 196
French Fries, 128, 130, 134, 142, 144
French Toast, 127
From the CUPboard, 78, 162-192
Fruit Breakfast Bar, 150
Fruit Jell-O, 150
Fruit Juice, 64, 120, 150, 156
Fruit Roll-Up, 150
Fruit Smoothie, 72, 91, 156
Fruit Syrup, 79, 81
Fudge, 66, 81, 125
Functional Diets, 39, 40
Gallbladder Disease, 30, 33
Garden Cress, 159
Garlic, 77, 132, 138, 159, 168, 180, 182, 183, 188-190, 192, 193
Gender, 23, 47, 85, 87
Genetic Predisposition, 40
Ghee Oil, 80
Global Reach Internet Productions, 14
Goat, 106, 120, 152, 157
Golf Ball (volume estimator), 57
Grains Food Group, 63-65, 82
Grape Seed Oil, 80
Grapefruit, 147
Grapes, 149
Green (-/Under), 55
Green Beans, 67, 77, 132
Green Chiles, 77, 188, 189, 192
Green Onions, 190

Grilled Pita Pizza (recipe), 164, 180, 181
Guacamole, 81, 140, 147
Guava, 148
Gynecological Problems, 33
Ham, 69, 126, 139, 152, 156
Hamburger, 126-129, 134, 142-144
Harris-Benedict Equation (rev.), 44, 85
Hazelnuts and Nuts, 153
Healthy Approach in Losing Weight, 28
Healthy Weight, 25, 28 36, 44, 47
Heart Disease, 30, 33, 34, 37, 38
Height, 23, 31, 36, 85, 87
Hicaco, 148
Honey, 81, 113, 133, 137
Hormonal and Neurological Changes, 85
Horseradish, 70, 80
Hot Dog, 129, 152
Hotcake, 93, 122, 126, 134
How Much Can I Eat?, 45, 46
How Much Do I NEED To Lose?, 35
How Much Do I WANT To Lose?, 35
How the CUPS diet® Works, 42
How Will I Stay Motivated?, 35
hummUs, 81, 156
Hunger, 40, 74, 83
Hyperlinks, 20
Hypertension, 30, 33
Hypothyroidism, 88
Ice Cream, 66, 123, 125, 130
Ideal Weight, 18, 35, 36, 56
Illnesses and Fevers, 88
Improved Weight Status Category, 38
International Users of the CUPS diet®, 3
Iodine, 86
Iowa Psychiatric Society, 17
Iowa State University, 16
Iphone, 21
Irregularly Shaped Portions, 60
Italian Roasted Potatoes (recipe), 164, 202, 203
Jackfruit, 149
Jam, 81, 151
Jamun Fruit
Jicama, 159

Jogging, 89
John M. De Castro, Dept. of Psych., 71
Joint Replacements, 6
Journal of Clinical Endocrinology and
    Metabolism, 73
Juice, 63, 64, 69, 70, 77, 92, 120, 150,
    156, 168, 186
Kale, 136, 159
Kempo Karate, 48
Ketchup, 80
Kiwifruit, 148
Kohlrabi (German turnips), 159
Kumquat, 149
KUPS for KIDS™, 194
Lamb, 69, 152
Lambert Adolphe Jacques Quetele, 31
Land of "thin", 25
Lean Body Mass, 87, 89
Leeks, 159
legUmes, 67, 161
Lemon, 70, 148, 168, 169, 184, 185, 187
Lentils (legUmes), 65, 67, 161
Lettuce, 96, 106, 155, 159, 168, 169
LFP - Low Fat Preferred, 64, 69, 79
Lime, 70, 77, 104, 148, 188, 189
Limit Eating at TV/Computer, 84
Liquor, 118
Liver Disease, 33
Lobster, 152
Loss of Muscle Tissue, 86
Lost Body Fluids, 86
Low Energy, 27
Low to Moderate Calorie Diet, 87
Lunch, 71, 74, 76, 90
Lunch Examples, 98-103
Lychee, 149
M - Meat, 63, 65, 69, 70, 75, 81, 82, 90,
    96, 117, 151, 152, 155
Malnutrition, 86
Mandarin Oranges, 148
Mandarin Sauce, 137
Mango, 77, 145, 147, 188, 189
Maple Syrup, 81, 126, 134
Margarine, 66, 80, 81

Marinara Pasta Sauce, 110, 122
Marmite, 81
Mascaro Family Recipes, 78, 162-192
Mascaro Health, Inc., 1
Mashed Potatoes, 60, 132, 161
Mayonnaise, 66, 81, 172, 173, 190, 191
Meals, 14, 23, 25, 28, 39, 41, 46, 49, 52,
    53, 56, 63-65, 67, 69, 71-74, 77, 78,
    83, 84, 90-116
Meals, Snacks, and Water, 71, 72, 74, 78
Measuring CUP Increments, 22, 41-44,
    46, 58, 60
Meat Spreads, 81
Mediterranean Potato Salad (recipe), 184
Melons, 146
Menstruation, 88
Metabolism, 8, 22, 40, 42-44, 46, 48, 71,
    73, 85-89
Mexican Pizza, 141
Milk, 8, 57, 64, 66, 72, 80, 91, 93, 94, 96,
    120, 153, 157, 166, 167, 170, 171, 178,
    179, 186, 187, 193
Milk Carton (volume estimator), 57
Mixed Drinks, 118
Molasses, 81
Mombin, 147
Mood Symptoms, 27
Morbid Obesity, 31, 33, 34
Morir Soñando (recipe), 163, 186, 187
Motivation, 19, 27, 35-38, 59, 194
Mozzarella Stick, 144
Muscle (mass) Tissue, 85-89
Mushrooms, 92, 110, 129, 136, 159, 163-
    165, 180, 181
Mustard, 70, 81, 137, 168
Mustard Greens, 159
My Account, 50, 54
My Daily Progress, 47, 50-52, 54,
Nachos, 141
Naseberry, 147
National Heart, Lung, and Blood
    Institute (NHLBI), 31, 87
National Institutes of Health, 34, 38
National Weight Control Registry, 72

Nectarine, 148
NEW USERS START HERE, 50, 52
Non-Lean Tissues, 89
Norepinephrine, 88
Normal Weight, 31, 33, 34, 36
N. Am. Assn. for the Study of Obesity, 72
Nutella, 81
Nutrition, 18, 19, 22, 23, 39, 40, 43, 48,
    65, 71, 153
Nuts, 66, 97, 106, 153, 157
Ø - **NO** Count Foods and Beverages, 65,
    70, 75, 84, 90, 158, 189
Oatmeal, 65, 87, 122, 126, 134, 157
Obese Class I, II, and III, 31, 33
Obesity, 6, 15, 17, 22, 27, 30-34, 72
Obesity Action Coalition, 17
Obesus, 26, 30
Obtaining your **AIM**, 45, 46
Oils/Fats, 79, 80, 169
Okra, 159
Old Chinese Proverb, 38
Olive Oil, 80, 106, 157, 168, 180-182, 184
Olives, 149, 185
Onion Rings, 128, 130
Onions, 77, 106, 155, 159, 160, 170-175,
    180-183, 188-190, 192, 193
Opuntia, 159
Orange Juice, 92, 186, 187
Orange, 64, 68, 76, 147
Orangelo, 147
Osteoarthritis, 30, 33
Overweight, 6, 8, 15, 22, 31-34
Oysters, 152
Pager (volume estimator), 57
Pancake, 93, 122, 126, 134
Papaya, 147
Parfait, 130. 132, 135
Parsnip, 160
Passion Fruit, 147
Pasta, 62, 64, 99, 110, 122, 138
Pastry, 66, 125, 171
PDF Files, 78, 90, 117
Peaches, 147
Peanut Butter, 81, 95

Peanut Oil, 80
Peanuts, 153
Pears, 147
Peas, 160, 170, 171
Pecans and Nuts, 153
Peewah, 149
Peppers, 160
Perla Nancy González Salazar, RD, 14, 90
Persimmon, 148
Phosphorus, 64
Physical Activity, 5, 6, 9, 19, 35, 40, 42,
    48, 51, 83, 86, 89
Pickles, 155, 159
Pie, 66, 125, 132
Pine Nuts, 153
Pineapple, 147, 178
Pintos, 140
Pistachios and Nuts, 135
Pitaya, 148
Pizza, 62, 102, 138, 141, 142, 154, 180
Plums, 148
Pomegranate, 147
Pomelo, 147
Popcorn, 111, 157
Popsicle, 157
Pork, 69, 137, 152, 163, 174, 175
Portable and Convenient, 18, 19
Portion, 5, 7, 8, 17, 22, 26, 30, 40, 42, 43,
    49, 57-59, 67, 69, 79, 117, 146-149
Pot Pie, 132, 133, 163, 170, 176, 177
Potato Salad, 144, 161, 163, 184, 185
Potatoes, 60, 67, 76, 98, 108, 132, 140,
    144, 161, 163, 170, 171, 182-185
Potsticker Sauce, 136, 137
Poultry, 63, 69, 152
Powdered Sugar, 81
Pregnant, 9, 31, 36
Progress Tracking Calendar, 47, 50
Protein, 64, 65, 71, 82, 83
Protein Drinks, 121
Psychiatrist, 16, 26
Psychological Aspects, 25-28, 30
Pudding, 102, 112, 125, 157
Pumpkin, 160

Pumpkin Seed Oil, 80
Questions, Comments, or Suggestions, 19, 196
Quince, 148
Radicchio, 160
Radishes, 160
Rambutan, 149
Realistic Goals, 84
Recipe for Weight Loss, 49
Recipes from the CUPboard, 78, 162-192
Record Your CUPS, 50-53, 56, 74, 78
Red (+/Over), 55
Report on Physical Activity & Health, 89
Respiratory Problems, 33, 89
Rhubarb, 160
Rice Bran Oil, 80
Roger Jones, 14
Running, 89
Rutabaga, 160
Safflower Oil, 80
Salad Dressing, 63, 77, 80, 102, 110, 133, 168, 169
Salads, 63, 64, 77, 101, 129, 133, 135, 139, 141, 163, 168, 169
Salsa, 70, 77, 80, 140
Salsa (recipe), 77, 163, 188, 189, 193
Sandwiches, 60, 69, 96, 100, 127-130, 133, 134, 139, 140, 142-144, 155
Sapote, 160
Satsumi Orange, 148
Sauce, 70, 79, 80, 110, 122, 138, 173, 195
Sausage, 69, 126, 134, 152
Save, 50
Scallions, 160, 184, 185
Seafood, 63, 137, 152
Seaweed, 160
Seeds, 153, 157
Self-Image, 27
Serving, 26, 42, 43
Sesame Oil, 80
Shallots, 160
Sheep, 120, 152
Shortening, 66, 80, 166, 167, 176, 177
Shrimp, 99, 109, 136, 137, 152

Shrimp Cocktail, 80
Sign In, 23, 46, 50
Sign Up, 23, 46
Sleep, 43, 83
Sleep Apnea, 33
Slowing the Digestive Process, 64
Smaller Plates, 84
Snacks, 41, 49, 53, 64, 71, 73, 74, 76, 82, 84, 90, 133, 135. 150, 155-157, 178
Examples, 111-116
Snack Pak, 100 Calorie, 157
Sorrels, 160
Soup, 103, 104, 116, 136, 139, 157, 192
Soursop, 146
Sour Cream, 66, 80, 143, 191, 192
Southern Iowa Mental Health Center, 16
Soy Sauce, 80, 137
Soybean Oil, 80
Spanish Version, 194
Special Food Category, 22, 23, 63-65, 67, 69, 70
Reminders, 65, 75, 90, 117
Spices and Herbs, 12, 70, 80, 83
Spinach, 160
Spinach Dip, 163, 190, 191
Spreads, 70, 79, 81, 123, 143
Spring Roll, 136, 157
Squash, 160
Starfruit, 148
Starvation, 86
Steak Sauces, 80
Stock Your Kitchen, 83
Strawberries, 72, 76, 91, 93, 108, 149
Strength Training, 86
Stress Related Hormones, 88
Stroke, 33, 37
Success Points, 38
Success Stories, 5, 29, 37, 42
Sugar, 67, 79, 81, 119, 122, 126, 166, 167, 178, 179
Sugar Beet Syrup, 81
Suggested Daily Amount, 79
Sunflower Oil, 80
Sweet and Sour Sauce, 80, 137, 143

Swimming, 89
Syrup, 79, 81, 93, 94, 126
Taco, 69, 128, 140, 141
    Taco Rico (recipe), 163, 189, 192, 193
    Taco Salads, 141
Tamarind Fruit, 149
Tangerines, 148
Target, 41, 44, 45, 47
Tea, 12, 70, 72, 76, 77, 91-95, 97-99, 119
Tennis Ball (volume estimator), 57
Terms Used in this Book, 22
Testosterone, 88
The Obesity Society, 17
Thirst, 74, 83
Three Fingers (volume estimator), 57
Thyroid, 86, 88
To Lose One Pound, 42
Toast, 92, 95-97, 127, 169
Tofu, 65, 136, 161
Tomatillo, 160
Tomato Juice, 70, 120
Tomatoes, 70, 77, 96, 106, 139, 155, 157, 160, 180, 188, 189, 193
Tortilla, 65, 77, 109, 122, 157, 192, 193
Tracking Calendar, 47, 50
Triiodothyronine (T3) & Thyroxin (T4), 88
Tuna, 104, 156
Turnips, 160
U of Alabama At Birmingham's Hosp., 34
U.S. Public Health Service Commissioned Corps, 74
Underweight, 31, 33
Univ. of Iowa Hospitals & Clinics, 17, 26
Unprocessed Foods, 39
Update Weekly Weight, 46, 47, 50-52
Update Weight, 46, 50
Updateable, 18
Users of **the CUPS diet**®, 2, 3
Using the CUPS diet, 52, 78
Using **the CUPS diet**®, 23, 31, 40, 44, 49
V8 Juice, 70, 120
VANITY (appearance/comfort), 35, 37
Vegemite, 81

Vegetables, 8, 23, 39, 63-65, 67, 70, 75, 77, 80-82, 84, 90, 99, 102, 103, 108, 110, 117, 120, 136, 154, 155, 157-161, 171, 183, 189, 190, 191
    Juice, 70, 120
    Oil, 80
Very Low Calorie Diets (VLCD), 86, 87
Vinegar, 81, 106, 168, 184
Visualize your Progress, 60, 83
Vitamins A and D, 64
Waffle, 94, 122
Walking, 5, 83, 89
Walnuts, 106, 135, 137, 153
Wasabi, 70, 81
Water, 5, 49, 52, 53, 60, 70-74, 76, 83, 84, 113, 121
Watercress, 160
Water Chestnuts, 159, 160, 190, 191
Website Access, 18, 23, 45, 49, 50
Weight Associated Health Risks, 9, 22, 27, 32, 35-38, 50, 51
Weight Lifting, 89
Weight Loss Goal, 9, 35, 37, 38
Weight Loss Results, 4, 19, 52, 74, 194
Weight Loss Tips, 19, 194
Weight Maintenance, 39
Weight Management, 22, 42, 43, 194
Weight Status Category, 31, 38
White Bean Dip, 157
White Sugar, 81, 178
WHO's World Health Statistics '12, 32
Wine, 57, 118, 168, 184
Within **AIM** Indicator, 54
Worcestershire Sauce, 70, 80, 168, 172
Wraps, 135, 141, 196
Wt. Associated Health Risks, 50 52
www.thecupsdiet.com, 1, 11, 16, 18, 19, 23, 24, 31, 37, 45, 46, 50-54, 194
Yams, 161
Yeast, 166, 167
Yogurt, 64, 125, 151, 158, 187
Yuca, 161
Zucchini, 160